ABRAHAM COLLES

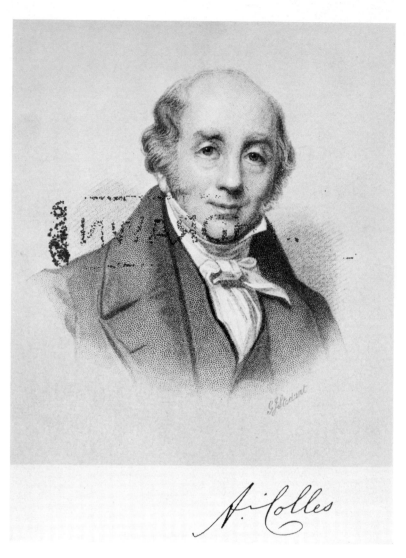

Abraham Colles (1773 – 1843)

[*Frontispiece*

ABRAHAM COLLES
1773—1843
Surgeon of Ireland

by

MARTIN FALLON

WILLIAM HEINEMANN MEDICAL BOOKS LTD

First Published 1972

© Martin Fallon 1972

ISBN 0 433 10110 5

In memoriam
CATHERINE O'BRIEN FALLON
1876–1937
and for
HAZEL, CHARLES, MICHAEL and NIGEL

Printed and bound in Great Britain by
R. J. Acford Ltd., Industrial Estate, Chichester, Sussex

Contents

List of Illustrations

Colles' Fracture—Cover.
Abraham Colles—Frontispiece.

The following illustrations appear between pages 130 and 131

1 William Colles of Kilcollen (1648–1719), eminent surgeon of Kilkenny. Great grandfather of Abraham Colles.

2 William Colles of Abbeyvale (1702–1770), distinguished citizen and Mayor of Kilkenny. Grandfather of Abraham Colles.

3 William Colles of Millmount (1745–1779); built Millmount in 1770, and married Mary Anne Bates in 1771. Father of Abraham Colles.

4 Millmount, Kilkenny, built by William Colles (1745–1779) in 1770. Photograph by courtesy of *The Kilkenny People.*

5 Abraham Colles as a young man. From a miniature in possession of Ronald M. Colles.

6 Abraham Colles' indenture certificate, 15 September 1790.

7 Abraham Colles' B.A. diploma, 9 April 1795. Trinity College, University of Dublin.

8 Abraham Colles' "Letters Testimonial" or Licence of the Royal College of Surgeons in Ireland, 24 September 1795.

9 Abraham Colles' Class Admission Tickets—
    1. Royal College of Surgeons in Ireland.
    2. Trinity College, Dublin.
    3. University of Edinburgh.

10 Dr. Steevens' Hospital, Dublin. Founded in 1720. Also a view of the Quadrangle of the Hospital looking east.

11 An eighteenth-century print of Trinity College, Dublin, showing the Library and its first Medical School, opened in 1711 (right foreground).

Acknowledgements

The author records his indebtedness and sincere thanks to:

The President, Vice-President, and Council of the Royal College of Surgeons in Ireland for access to the College records, and also for a grant to meet publication costs. The President of the College, Mr. Francis A. Duff, for the Foreword.

Members of the Colles family—

Ronald M. Colles, Captain A. C. Colles, R.N., Commander Sir Dudley Colles, K.C.B., K.C.V.O., R.N., Mrs. John Hyde-Thomson, Mrs. George Lucas, Christopher Colles McCready, Richard Colles Johnson, the Venerable Alexander Colles Nevill, Gerald E. Nevill, W. M. Colles, Oliver Lloyd, Mrs. Kendal Dixon, Mrs. Brian Clark, Mrs. Margaret Moore, Thomas Malcolm Colles Moore, and Mrs. Randolph Taylor for generously placing family records at his disposal.

Professor J. D. H. Widdess, Professor R. B. McDowell, Dr. Harry O'Flanagan, Mrs. Angela Butler, Professor Arthur Chance, Rt. Rev. H. R. McAdoo, Rev. Canon A. W. R. Camier, The officers of the College Historical Society of Trinity College, Dublin, and of the Speculative Society of Edinburgh, Mrs. Eileen Lambert, Mrs. Claire Murphy, Mrs. Margaret Phelan, Dr. James H. Spencer, Mr. John Corcoran, Mrs. Jill Martin, for various items of information from their records.

Major Adam Tilp-Zielinski, Miss Doreen Power, The Editor of *Surgery, Gynecology, and Obstetrics*, The Editor of the *Kilkenny People*, for photographs.

Professor J. W. L. Adams for a translation of Colles' M.D. Thesis.

My secretary, Miss Patricia Duncan, for cheerfully undertaking the onerous task of preparation of my manuscript, and Mrs. Lillian L. Chaplin for its final typescript.

My colleague and neighbour, Professor G. P. Henderson for his expert assistance in the correction of the proofs.

Foreword

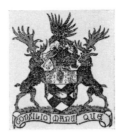

Under its Royal Charter, dated February 11th, 1784, the Royal College of Surgeons in Ireland was entrusted with the responsibility of maintaining the standards of surgical practice, and of establishing a liberal and extensive system of surgical education. To implement this, the Schools of Surgery were set up. As a result the College has been able to provide both a basic medical education and post graduate training facilities which would equip the young surgeon to become a master of his craft with the necessary scientific knowledge to look to and expand the horizon of clinical surgery.

In striving to fulfil these objectives the College, loyally supported by its professors teaching in many disciplines, has attracted students not only from these islands but from all over the world. Outstanding amongst them was Abraham Colles, appointed professor of anatomy and surgery in 1804. He had the distinction of being twice elected as president of the College. As a teacher, he was outstanding. Introducing his system of topographical anatomy, he was the first to develop the concept of surgical anatomy. He dominated the field of surgical education during the early part of the nineteenth century. His skill as a surgical observer is acknowledged all over the world by the acceptance by his colleagues of the fracture which bears his name and which he so accurately described in the Edinburgh medical and surgical Journal in 1814.

The era in which he lived was exciting. It covered the later Napoleonic years followed by the period of the rapid expansion. It was the starting point of explosive advance in scientific knowledge that gathered momentum during the nineteenth century.

Martin Fallon, after many years of detailed research into the life and times of Colles, draws a portrait full of warmth and interest of this master surgeon of Ireland. The publication of this excellent biography will be fitting recognition of the bicentenary of the birth of Colles on 23rd July, 1773.

Francis A. Duff

President, Royal College of Surgeons in Ireland

Preface

In the early decades of the nineteenth century a remarkable group of clinicians appeared in the Irish capital, who formed the "Irish" or "Dublin" School, which for a short while challenged the supremacy of Edinburgh as the leading medical centre in these Islands. Nothing like this ever happened before in Ireland; it has not happened since. Leading this group were Cheyne, Graves, Corrigan, and Stokes—a quartet which Edinburgh even in its greatest days could not match at any one time. Their surgical counterpart was Abraham Colles, who stood out among his contemporaries with a pre-eminence akin to theirs. Colles was then Ireland's leading surgeon. His name is inextricably linked with the dramatic rise of the Surgeons' School of the Royal College of Surgeons in Ireland. One of the earliest licentiates of its School, he became its greatest professor.

That century opened with a new profession of surgery whose members a few decades before ranked only as tradesmen, and were "below the salt". They henceforth took their places as full and responsible members of a liberal profession. Abraham Colles in his own land did more than anyone else to make the profession of surgery respectable. His remarkable ability as a teacher and brilliant anatomist made his School famous. As a surgeon he was shrewd and practical, and his common-sense approach gained for him an enormous surgical practice.

But it is not solely on his academic and professional eminence, nor on his publications and eponyms that his fame rests; he had also that quality which his fellow-countryman, Edmund Burke, described as the "chastity of honour", an honesty and modesty rare in that or in any other generation. It is this combination of gifts which earned for him and his country a more than respectable place in the history of surgery.

Martin Fallon.

". . . my venerated friend and teacher . . . this remarkable man and eminent surgeon."

"Were I the biographer of Mr. Colles I might enlarge on the many qualities of his mind, on the independence of his character, his boldness of thought, his warmth and largeness of heart, and his unquenchable zeal in the practice and teaching of his profession. It is only when we lose a great possession that we are able to estimate its full value. But it is a privilege allowed to the good and wise, that their example, which is in one sense their spirit remains after them. Clear in his conviction, as to what was right and steadfast to do and to teach only that which he thought was right, Mr. Colles gave to Irish surgery a great impetus and a lustre which it cannot lose."

William Stokes

(1854)

"Diseases of the Heart and Aorta"

CHAPTER 1

History—Fact and Fancy

"We are, all of us, Children of our Fathers. What we are is in part only of our own making, the greater part of ourselves has come down to us from the past. What we know and what we think is not a new fountain gushing fresh from the barren rock of the unknown at the stroke of the rod of our own intellect, it is a stream which flows by us and through us, fed by the far-off rivulets of long ago."

Sir Michael Foster (1901).

Surgery is the oldest branch of the healing art, as old as man and as old as trauma. Injury was a tangible thing demanding attention, and early man's first reaction was to protect the injured area from the influence of external forces or agents. He applied a dressing to a wound, using perhaps a leaf or shrub, and experience taught him which of these was best. He stopped haemorrhage by a variety of agents; he learnt that cobwebs were useful, the North American Indian found that snow was efficient, and the early Egyptian knew the benefit of applying raw steak to wounds. Primitive man sutured wounds, using bone needles and thorns, and for larger wounds he used the heated spear as a cautery. Splints were applied to fractured limbs and leeches were used to remove surplus blood. This approach was practical and rational, and its practitioner, whom we can now call the surgeon, naturally had his talents employed in other activities in the tribe, such as branding slaves, gelding animals, and drawing teeth.

But with medical or internal disease, primitive man was not so lucky. The existence of what we now term "natural causes" was not admitted, and all diseases were regarded as being due to a malevolent influence exercised by the gods or a human enemy.

Medicine and religion were early associates. The first physician, the Egyptian Imhotep (2980 B.C.) was later raised to the status of a god and the early medical papyri showed evidence of magical practice with charms and incantations. It should be noted that in early Egypt there was no division in the healing art; medicine and surgery were practised by the same individual. Nor did the Greeks make any distinction. The great schism in the healing art took place with the Arabs between the seventh and thirteenth centuries, to emerge again in the hauteur of the Paris faculty centuries later.

To the Greeks we owe the separation of medicine from the realm of magic and the tyranny of the gods. They came to base their practice upon observation and investigation, although this occurred in the later years of their glorious epoch. Hippocrates, the Father of Medicine, who lived in the fifth century B.C., first taught that disease was subject to and explainable by natural laws. Hippocrates laid down the ethics of the healing art, made many contributions to both medicine and surgery, and in practice was skilled in both. But the teaching of the Greeks did not entirely eliminate the association of medicine with religion, and even in later centuries the early Christian church did not allow medicine to develop as a separate discipline. The bishops and monasteries granted and controlled licences to practice medicine, a system continued under the reformed church. An Act of Henry VIII in 1534 empowered the Archbishop of Canterbury to grant degrees in medicine as well as in other faculties. The "Lambeth" M.D.,* however, was not registerable under the Medical Act of 1858, and since that date has been granted only occasionally as a decoration and then only to those already on the Medical Register.

Historians tell us that the "Green Isle" was first inhabited by the Fomorians—gloomy giants of the sea, and later by the Firbolgs, who were described as dark, short and plebeian. Next in possession were the Tuatha De Danann, who were a superior race, semi-divine in their arts of magic and wizardry. The first medical figure to emerge from the mists of Irish antiquity was Dian Cecht, often referred to as the "Irish Asclepius" or God of Healing. Nuadhat, chief of the De Danann,

*Last bestowed in 1880.

lost his hand in battle with Firbolgs at Moytura in 487 B.C., and as the deformity would debar him from kingship, Dian Cecht had a hand fashioned in silver and fitted to the king. The hand was beautiful to behold and we are told was capable of movement and even of sensation! It represents the first example of the limb fitter's art and in recent times has been adopted as part of the crest of the Medical Corps of the Irish Army.

The next invaders were the Celts, about 350 B.C. They were tall and red-blond of hair. Originally spread over central Europe, they migrated west—those from France invaded and conquered Britain, those from Spain conquered Ireland, and are referred to as the Milesians. They were warring tribes and the important ones founded kingdoms. We next read of Fingin, physician to Connor Mac Nessa, king of Ulster, about the beginning of the Christian era. When the king was wounded in the head by a missile from a sling, Fingin stitched the wound with threads of gold to match the king's hair. Surgical progress continued, and in the great days of Fionn Mac Cumhail we are told that the skin of an ewe was fixed to the skinless part of one of his warriors. The graft took so well that a fleece of wool had to be shorn periodically from its surface! Those warriors apparently engaged in fierce combat only by day, and after a truce at sundown, they dressed one another's wounds, shared provisions, medicated baths, and also one another's company. This chivalrous action, in the Gaelic term *comraind legis*, or "impartial treatment of the wounded", was a primitive form of Red Cross organisation.

The Celts brought with them their own customs and code of laws—The Brehon Laws, which were set out centuries before the birth of Christ and represent the most ancient code in Europe. The medical clauses only concern us here—the sick were provided with special accommodation and protected from fools and female scolds. The physician ranked high in the Council of State and his payment varied according to the social grade of the patient. A referee was provided should any dispute arise between patient and physician. The negligent physician was fined. The aggressor in quarrels resulting in injury, had to pay compensation to the injured man and be responsible for payment of the physician and other attendants' fees. Special sections of the code dealt with the care of the insane. The Brehon code of laws, although modified on the introduction of Christianity, persisted until the reign of James I.

These warring tribes and kingdoms of the Celts extended their activities, and their galleys were dreaded on the coasts of Britain and Gaul; the Romans never invaded Ireland. But all this was changed in 432 A.D. when Patrick, a citizen of the Empire, arrived with the Christian faith and opened up the island to Latin civilisation and the culture of Rome, which, though the Empire died, survived in the Church. The change was immediate and profound. The new monasteries poured forth missionaries to spread Christianity to neighbouring lands. The arts and learning thrived, silver and gold were worked into beautiful objects, and the manuscripts that have come down to us are among the world's treasures. This was Ireland's Golden Age, and in the words of an English parliamentarian, "Ireland alone almost for seven centuries maintained the culture of the western world".

The monasteries alone provided medical care. In the Benedictine rule we read, "The care of the sick is to be placed above and before every other thing, as if indeed Christ were being directly served in waiting upon them. The infirmarian must be thoroughly reliable, known for his piety and diligence, and solicitude for his charge. Baths to be provided for the sick as often as they need them." Thus spiritual and temporal care became closely linked, and there is evidence that in Ireland the bishops alone granted licences to those allowed to practise the healing art. Some of the monks appear to have had some surgical skill. St. Bricin in 637 A.D. performed a decompression operation on the skull of a wounded warrior. We are told that the "brain of forgetfulness" was removed. While away in the monastery of Monte Cassino, St. Benedict removed a bladder stone from the German monarch Henry II in 1000 A.D. and the king survived for twenty-four years. The famous woodcut of that operation scene suggests that this was performed by the suprapubic route.

Care of the tonsure was naturally an important feature in monastic life, and this duty was performed by the lower order of monks, the lay servants, or *barbitonsores*, who, in addition, became expert in the simple surgical procedures of bloodletting, tooth drawing, reduction of fractures and dislocations, the opening of abscesses, and the stitching of wounds. By an edict of the Council of Tours in 1163, *ecclesia abhorret a sanguine*, the monastic orders were forbidden to take part in any surgical procedures involving blood and the monasteries then cast out their lay brothers and servants who practised the surgical and barber's art. Beginnings, as Carlyle reminds us, are formidable things. Those outcasts from the monasteries whom we may now call the barber-surgeons, set up little businesses of their own in the various towns and cities. They were simple tradesmen, and like other tradesmen, displayed recognition signs over their shops to be recognised by an illiterate populance. The barber's pole represents the phlebotomist's staff which the patient grasped during bloodletting, the red stripe represents the fillet or bandage placed above the elbow to contract the veins, and the white stripe the bandage placed over the elbow later. From the pole was suspended a basin which in practice collected the blood, untold quantities of which flowed during the many centuries when this form of therapy was a prominent feature in the treatment of many diseases. The barber-surgeon had no standards or limits to his activities, ranging from man mid-wife to sow gelder. Many travelled throughout the land, setting up booths and stalls in the market place during fairs and gatherings, advertising their skills and practising their many and pain-producing arts on a credulous populace. Some were better educated and attracted apprentices, the better ones attached themselves to the households of chieftains and kings, and accompanied their masters to the wars—Lanfranc, Guy de Chauliac, John of Arderne, Ambrose Paré, were of these, and upheld the best traditions of their craft. In Ireland, the barber-surgeon was a sort of general medical practitioner, competing with the apothecaries and the "hereditary" physicians (the O'Lees, the O'Hickeys, the O'Sheils, and the O'Callenans) who had the medical care of ancient Irish families.

For two centuries, 800–1014 A.D., the Norsemen invaded and ravished the Irish coasts and countryside. They were finally beaten off at Clontarf in 1014, and this date also was the end of

Ireland's heroic age. Thereafter followed a period of political confusion and difficulties between the Pope and his Irish Church. One of the minor differences was the shape and extent of the Irish monastic tonsure, which did not conform to the universal standards of the Church. Perhaps, after all, the Church was missing its barbers!

Henry II arrived with his Normans in Ireland in 1172—whether by invitation of its rulers or by a concession of the Pope to reform the Church, or to the rescue of a Dark Rosaleen, historians do not guide us. The next eight centuries of Irish history are nothing more than a continuous struggle between these Norman English invaders, and native Ireland, with politics and religion taking up a disproportionate space of Irish history. These centuries had left ragged wounds in the shaping of the national character of Ireland, and equally ugly scars in the conscience of England.

In 1172 Henry II made a grant of the city of Dublin to his "men of Bristol". Twenty years later their charter made reference to the Dublin guilds, and of the sixteen hundred names inscribed on their rolls not a single Irish name appears. All were without exception Norman names. On October 18, 1446 Henry VI granted a Royal Charter to the Barber-Surgeons of Dublin as a reward for their services to his soldiery. The establishment of this guild in Dublin was the earliest recognition by ruling monarchy of the craft of surgery in these islands, for the London guild was not incorporated until later in the same century (1461), and our brethren in Edinburgh had to wait for their Seill of Cause till the following century (1505). The first master of the Dublin guild was a Bristol man, but in what spirit of repentence he and his brother wardens selected the Blessed Mary Magdalene as their patron saint, contemporary records do not reveal. The probable explanation is that they were allotted a chantry in the Church of Saint Mary Magdalene which then stood within the precincts of the Hospital of Saint John, outside the New Gate of the city. Of the twenty-five guilds in the city the Barbers' guild ranked fourth, being preceded by the Trinity guild of merchants, the tailors, and the smiths. Although described as a guild of Barbers it was specifically stated that it was "for the promotion and exercise of the art of chirurgery", and Cameron is satisfied that in the fifteenth century the terms barber and chirurgeon were exactly equivalent. It is noteworthy that the guild was empowered to admit women to all their rights and privileges. The charter of Henry VI is no longer extant and Berry considers that it was lost in 1754 when given out for translation. Fortunately its contents are restated in the preamble to Elizabeth's charter, which can now be seen in the library of Trinity College, Dublin.

A century later there were surgeons in Dublin who were not members of the Barbers' guild, and Queen Elizabeth found it necessary to grant a new charter in 1577—"To blend, join and reduce the said distinct and separate societies of barbers and chirurgeons, into one body that in close aggregate and connected fellowship the art and science of chirurgery might flourish as well in theory as in practice and would greatly conduce to and be a means of perfecting learning and exercising the art aforesaid and assisting both themselves and their present and future apprentices". It is clear, then, that in the age of Queen Elizabeth hair cutting and dressing and shaving were not practised as a distinct mystery by the Barbers. Up to 1642 the Dublin Barber-Surgeons' guild were using as their Arms almost an exact copy of those granted to the London Company. Three years later (1645) they were granted their own Coat of Arms for their loyalty and services to Charles I. This was emblazoned on their hearses so that "their funerals could be celebrated after the most decent manner befitting their quality". The Ulster King-at-Arms referred to them as a profession. The guild of Barber-Surgeons met in their own Hall over the Pole Gate in the city wall in Bride Street, and were also allotted one of the chapels in Christ Church Cathedral. Later, the guild shared the Tailors' Hall with other city guilds.

In 1687 the Dublin Corporation was dissolved on refusing to admit Roman Catholics to their privileges and offices, and when reconstituted it was necessary to issue new charters to the guilds. The new charter of James II (1687) was one of the many stupid acts of that hapless monarch. In addition to the barber-surgeons, the apothecaries and the periwig-makers were now added to the guild, and the surgeons, being hopelessly

outnumbered in this motley group, began to draw apart. At
the beginning of the eighteenth century there were many
surgeons in Dublin not members of the confraternity, e.g. army
surgeons, men of liberal education who studied at universities
at home and abroad, and others who had served apprenticeship to surgeons of good standing. In practice, there was free
trade in surgery at that time. A pamphlet, now in the National
Library of Ireland, published about 1703, was addressed to both
the Irish House of Lords and House of Commons, and reads—

> "The present Corporation in this City is composed of Barbers,
> Surgeons, Apothecaries and Peruke-Makers, which (instead
> of Encouraging the true Professors of Surgery) is a refuge of
> Empiricks, Impudent Quacks, Women, and other idle
> Persons, who quit the Trades to which they were bred, and
> wherein they might be useful to the Commonwealth, to
> undertake a Profession whereof they are entirely ignorant,
> to the ruine of their Fellow Subjects.
>
> There is not any Person (tho of the most Infamous Character)
> who cannot obtain his Freedom of the Corporation, by Vertue
> whereof, the meanest Brother assumeth the Liberty, and it is
> sufficient Recommendation for him to Practise Surgery,
> with as much Authority as the most Experienced Surgeon.
>
> There are in the Corporation at least Ten Barbers, etc. for
> one Surgeon, so that it is impossible for the Surgeons to
> make any Regulation, because they must inevitably be out-
> voted by the Majority of the others.
>
> There is not the least Affinity between Surgery, Peruke-
> Making and the Feat or Craft of Barbery, it not being
> necessary for a Surgeon to know how to make a Peruke or
> Cut Hair, nor is it part of a Barber's or Peruke-Makers Trade,
> to perform any Operation in Surgery" . . . (see Appendix).

Between 1702 and 1714, surgeons who were independent of
the Barber-Surgeons' guild, called upon the Irish Parliament to
separate the surgeons from the barbers, apothecaries, and
periwig-makers, but their petition failed. In 1716 the Barber-
Surgeons' guild had correspondence with Thomas Proby, the
Surgeon-General, in reference to his practising surgery without

being a member of the fraternity. Proby wrote polite replies, expressing his doubts that all the surgeons in Dublin could be combined in one body owing to its peculiar constitution. In 1741 the Barber-Surgeons offered the freedom of their guild to the president, censors and fellows of the Royal College of Physicians, and proposed a conjoint examination by physicians and surgeons as the mode of admission to their guild, but their suggestions were not adopted by the physicians. In 1745 the apothecaries separated from the Barber-Surgeons' guild and formed their own guild of St. Luke. This was the last guild to be constituted in Dublin and its members do not seem to have been very popular, as a verse published anonymously in 1767 reads—

"See, where the proud Apothecaries drive,
Who most by fraud and imposition thrive,
Whose monstrous bills immoderate wealth procure
For drugs that kill as many as they cure,
Well are they placed the last of all the rout,
For they're the men we best can do without."

When the apothecaries left the Barber-Surgeons' guild, the surgeons themselves took no further interest in the parent guild, nor did they consider themselves subject to its control. Although in practice the foundation of the Royal College of Surgeons (1784) had separated the surgeons completely from the barbers, yet nominally they remained united until the city guilds disappeared in consequence of the passing of the Municipal Corporations (Ireland) Act in 1840.

We must remember that the struggles of the Irish surgeons and their British colleagues to establish themselves as a liberal profession, owe their inspiration to the establishment in 1731 at Paris of the Académie Royale de Chirurgie, with Georges Mareschal its founder as first president. This freed the surgeons from the long-borne domination by the physicians of the faculty, bringing the healing art back to the ancient unity which it enjoyed in the days of Greece, as symbolised in the medal struck by the Academy in which appear the figures of Fernel and Paré, physician and surgeon of the Renaissance, above the prophetic legend—*La médicine rendue à son unité primitive.* The

Royal Academy of Surgery established in 1731 survived only some fifty years, as with other academies of Royal foundation it was suppressed by the Convention, to be replaced in the year III of the Republic (1792) by the Écoles de Santé. Under the Bourbon restoration these became the École de Médicine (1820) and the handsome building which in the last quarter of the eighteenth century (1776) had been erected to house Mareschal's creation is to-day the École de Médicine of Paris. Mareschals' Academy served as the prototype for the Royal Colleges later to be chartered in these islands, at Edinburgh 1778, Dublin 1784, and London 1800.

Georges Mareschal, one of surgery's immortals, has a special place in the affection of Irishmen. The story of this orphan boy who rose to be chief surgeon to two kings of France, has often been related, but by none better than my friend, the late William Doolin. In the sixteenth and seventeenth centuries the defeated Irish soldiers were not accorded the traditional honours meted out to the vanquished, and as they were not prepared to serve as slaves, they took leave of their land and all they loved. When the heartrending scenes and the wails of their womenfolk subsided at the quay-side, they sailed away into the mists, never to return, to fight again under the lilies of France. It is estimated that 25,000 of these left Ireland and ever since, in song and story, their flight has gained for them the sobriquet of the "Wild Geese". John Marshall of Limerick was one of these, who after the 1641 Rebellion escaped to France to join the armies of Louis XIII during the Thirty Years War. Wounded, with loss of an arm fighting the Spaniards on the field at Recroy, he retired and became a small innkeeper at Calais, and in due course married a widow. Their son, Georges, was born in 1658. This young boy, losing both his parents at the age of thirteen, set out alone on the long walk to Paris, with a total capital of less than £4, and on arrival there was to take another long walk through the pages of the history of surgery.

In 1765 an Act of the Irish Parliament established the County Infirmaries Board—the first surgical examining body in Ireland. All surgeons appointed to the newly established infirmaries had to pass an examination in anatomy and surgery; the

Surgeon-General, and the surgeons of Dr. Steevens' and Mercer's Hospitals acting as examiners. More candidates were rejected for not having fulfilled their indentures than for lack of knowledge of surgery. Although styled "surgeons", most of their practice in the infirmaries was essentially medical. The Board first met at the Music Hall in Fishamble Street, a building immortalised by Handel, who first produced his *Messiah* there in 1742 to raise funds for Mercer's Hospital. The County Infirmaries Board ceased to function after 1796, when its duties as examiners were taken over by the Royal College of Surgeons in Ireland.

In 1765, Sylvester O'Halloran (1728–1807) the distinguished Limerick surgeon and littérateur, made recommendations for the advancement of surgical education in Ireland, which were published as an appendix to his book on gangrene and sphacelus. After referring to the superior status of surgery in France, he writes of the surgical practice pertaining at home—

"Indeed the daily injuries committed by ignorant quacks call loudly for reformation. A slight sore, a fixt pain, rheumatic, nay paralitic complaints, are causes sufficient for these gentry to salivate: the mercury is poured on in such profuse quantities as frequently to destroy—in general to impoverish the constitution, and make the sick of little use after. Nay, so violent are their common purges, that the prudence of the apothecary is what preserves the patient. And what else can be expected, when wretches who can scarce write, seem to amuse themselves with the most drastic drugs with impunity? Nay, there are not wanting instances in a more exalted state, where men of greater character than abilities have absolutely destroyed the sick through the grossest ignorance! To prevent such fatal mistakes for the future and to preserve the vigour of our commonalty, already greatly degenerated, the following proposals for the advancement of our surgery, are submitted to public consideration:—

(1) That a decent and convenient edifice be erected in the capital, and three professorships founded—one for anatomy, a second for the disorders of surgery and midwifery, and the third for the operations of surgery:

and that each do give a course of lectures in succession every winter free to all people.

(2) That an exact list be taken through the kingdom of all the reputable surgeons, with their names and places of abode; that no others presume to practise surgery, much less to perform capital operations; and that all young surgeons from time to time be interdicted practice, till they shall procure a faculty of their abilities, signed by the above professors, or their successors.

(3) In order to procure this, the candidate or candidates must by written notice apply for a public examination and this to be published before the exhibition which should be from twelve to three o'clock. That this hold for three days; the first entirely for anatomy, the second for disorders of surgery, and, if a candidate for midwifery, for this also; and the third to finish, with performing all the operations of surgery on a body, with their apparatus and bandaging. When a proper faculty signed by the professors, is given to the candidate, to which, if some little honor were annexed, it might add greater stimulus to the young students.

(4) That this course be attended with no kind of expense to the candidate, and that it be free to all Irishmen *only*, without distinction; genius being unconfined to principle or party, and such narrower considerations being worthier of a little republic of Ragusa, than the representatives of a powerful kingdom. And that the number be by no means limited, because the more surgeons of eminence the better will the public be served.

(5) That a printed list be published annually of the registered surgeons, and men-midwives of the kingdom, with their places of abode, signed by the professors: by which means the public will, *as heretofore*, know where to apply for certain relief."

O'Halloran, who studied at Leiden and Paris, was founder of and surgeon to the County Limerick Infirmary, and was described as "the tall, thin doctor, in his quaint French dress, with his gold-headed cane, beautiful Parisian wig and cocked hat". He did not hesitate to revive and use the ancient Gaelic motto of his family—*Lothaim agus marhbaim,** despite its unsuitability for a surgeon, and lived long enough to see his ideas on surgical reform put into practice. Mapother rightly stresses the influence that O'Halloran's views had on the evolution of Irish surgery. O'Halloran was made an honorary member of the Dublin Society of Surgeons in 1780 and of the Royal College of Surgeons in Ireland in 1786.

In 1773 and again in 1775, Samuel Croker-King, later the first president of the College, petitioned the Irish Parliament for an act regulating the practice of surgery, but the bills were not proceeded with: and William Dease in the introduction to his books (1778 and 1782) also stressed the necessity for a Royal Charter for the Irish surgeons. Meanwhile the Dublin Society of Surgeons was founded in 1780 under the presidency of Henry Morris, surgeon to Mercer's Hospital, and renowned for his successful removal of a bladder stone weighing some $15\frac{1}{2}$ ounces. This Society, of nineteen members, met frequently in city taverns and dined together quarterly. In this convivial atmosphere there is, understandably, no record that any papers were read or scientific business transacted. A committee of the Society, however, was formed to agitate for a charter, and in 1780 they resolved—"That it is the opinion of this Committee that a Royal Charter, dissolving the preposterous and disgraceful union of the surgeons of Dublin with the barbers, and incorporating them separately and distinctly, upon liberal and scientific principles, would highly contribute not only to their own emolument and the advancement of the profession in Ireland, but to the good of society in general, by cultivating and diffusing surgical knowledge". A petition was presented to the Lord Lieutenant in 1781, which was referred by him to the Barber-Surgeons for their comment. The latter recited the various charters upon which their privileges rested, and protested that they could not consent to any request of the petitioners which might interfere with their rights, describing themselves as "faithful and loyal Protestant subjects of the best of kings".

* I wound and I kill.

Fortunately "the best of kings" (George III) was then sane, and a Royal Charter was granted on the 11th February 1784, and the Royal College of Surgeons in Ireland came into being. Appropriately, they first met in the Lying-In Hospital (Rotunda), the oldest maternity hospital in these islands. Grasping their baby charter they went forth into a turbulent world (not forgetting to tip the hospital porter and to give a piece of silver to the matron) without prospects or patrons and without a home.   These surgical pioneers, Protestant and Papist, Loyalist and Nationalist alike, were true surgical *Sinn Feiners*.* None of these men ever appear to have been at a university, but each could anticipate Winston Churchill's quizzical remarks to new graduates of a later century†— "Unlike you, I have no technical and no university education, and have just had to pick up a few things as I went along"! Ignored by the Physicians and the University and receiving no help from colleagues at home or abroad, they set their course alone. They appointed professors, who at first lectured in their own homes without any fee, and five years later (1789) established their own School. In the following year, Abraham Colles entered that Surgeons' School as a registered pupil.

---

* Sinn Fein—ourselves alone.

† M.I.T. Boston 1949.

CHAPTER 2

The Colles Family

It is perhaps but natural that some little taint of vain
glory should creep into a thing of this kind,
as, for instance, when one knows that he comes
of a long and virtuous line.

                    Benevenuto Cellini.

The Colles family tree is of considerable antiquity and appears
from the earliest records to have been first established in
Somerset. Its early spelling Collé suggests French or Anglo-
Norman origin. A distinguished member of the family during
the earlier part of the fifteenth century was Walter Colles,
Precentor and Chancellor of Exeter Cathedral and Constable
of Bordeaux. He negotiated various treaties with France on
behalf of King Henry V and King Henry VI of England. In
the Parish Church of Pitminister there are elaborate monuments to Humphrey Colles, John Colles and John Colles
(junior). These, father, son and grandson, were all in turn
High Sheriffs of the County of Somerset in the sixteenth and
seventeenth centuries.

About the middle of the thirteenth century an off-shoot of
this Somerset family settled in Worcestershire and subsequently
in Warwickshire and neighbouring counties. For several
centuries thereafter these were important people and inter-
married with the great families of the midlands. Between 1298
and 1341 a member of the Colles family represented the city of
Worcester in Parliament on fifteen occasions. In 1515, one
Boniface Colles, secretary to the Bishop of Worcester, brought
from Rome the cardinal's hat and accompanying bull for
Wolsey. The hat was placed on Wolsey's head during an imposing ceremony in Westminster Abbey. The Pope (Leo X)
and the cardinal highly praised Boniface for his part in the

ceremony and a pleased Henry VIII gave him £66 13s. 4d. for his services.

An important branch of the Worcestershire family stems from Richard Colles (1448) (see Appendix) of Powick in Suckley, from which by tradition if not in fact the Irish branch of the family has descended. Richard's grandson, William Colles, (1495–1558) of Leigh is buried in Leigh Parish Church and in the same church there are elaborate monuments to the latter's son, Edmund Colles (1530–1606) and grandson, William Colles (1560–1615). Leigh Manor adjacent to Leigh Church belonged to the Abbots of Pershore and at the dissolution of the monasteries was acquired by Edmund Colles, first as a tenant and later by purchase. This Edmund Colles was an important person locally, and he also acquired extensive lands and property at Lulsley, Grimley and Suckley, which on his death were passed to his son, William. Of the original Leigh Manor only its magnificent tithe barn now remains. The Colles family fortunes now appear to have disintegrated rapidly, and some years after the death of William Colles in 1615 the lands were sold by his son and heir, Edmund Colles, the younger, to the Deveraux family. Edmund Colles, the last of the Leigh family, "being loaded with debts which like a snowball from Malvern Hill, gathered increase", was a notorious character if local legends are to be believed. Once, when deeply in debt, he heard that his greatest friend, who lived at Cradley, had gone to Worcester to receive a large sum of money. Colles planned to attack him on his return and escape with the booty unrecognised in the dark. The friend, however, was well armed, and drawing his broadsword he cut at his unknown assailant and drove him off. When he arrived at Cradley he found a bloody hand gripping his horse's bridle. He was horrified at discovering the signet ring of his bosom friend on one of the fingers. The following day he rode over to Leigh Court with the hand and the ring, and was told that Colles was very ill in bed, but insisted on being admitted to his room. Colles, taxed with the crime, confessed his guilt, and bursting into tears, prayed for mercy, which was magnanimously granted. A tradition also exists that this Edmund Colles murdered a man and bricked up his body in a cellar of the farm. When fleeing across the Teme with his wife and family after the deed, his children were drowned, but he and his lady escaped. There was also a legend that his ghost used to drive a coach and four fiery steeds down the hill at midnight, dash over the tithe barn and disappear into the Teme. But it was not the dissipation of Edmund Colles, the younger, alone, that led to the loss of the family fortunes and estates, and the disappearance of the family from the midlands in the seventeenth century. To discover the probable reason, we must call to mind the state of the time between 1641 and 1660. We learn from the history of that very troubled period that practically all the noble and gentle families of Worcestershire and adjoining counties espoused the interest of Charles I in the Civil War, and devoted their means as well as their lives to his cause. For this reason, as well as the heavy fines imposed on all Royalists by Parliament, and through being unable to get their rents, they were compelled to sell their estates. Still, they looked forward hopefully to being in some degree requited for all their losses and sacrifices on the accession of Charles II. In this anticipation they were very shortly to be deceived. Charles, after his restoration, turned his back on those friends of his father, and declined absolutely to assist them in any way. The great majority of the suffering cavaliers found no remedy for their losses by any process of law, as the Act of Indemnity put a stop to any suit of law they might have instituted. They bitterly felt the statute to be, as they expressed it, an act of indemnity for the King's enemies and of oblivion for his friends. Thus they found themselves finally "abandoned to the comfort of an irreparable but honourable ruin". That the Colles family was far from being the only one which suffered from the effects of the Civil War and the subsequent financial troubles, is clearly revealed by the fact that in Worcestershire alone the names of approximately one hundred and thirty county families recorded in the Herald's visitation of 1634 are absent from that of 1682. Sir Walter Deveraux, Bart., who acquired the Colles estates sometime between 1660 and 1682, was a cousin of the Earl of Essex, who was in supreme command of Parliament's army in the Civil War and, like him, it may be assumed that he was a Parliamentarian, which is confirmed by the consideration that had he been a Royalist he could hardly have been left the means to maintain an estate, and much less to purchase one.

There can be little doubt that William Colles, who started the Irish branch of the family, came of this family of Leigh, in Worcestershire. The crest of the Colles family in Ireland is that of Colles of Leigh, as evidenced in the funeral entry of Charles Colles (1610–1685) in the Ulster King-at-Arms office in Dublin Castle, and it was to the English midlands that the early members of the Irish family returned. Exhaustive enquiries by John A. Purefoy Colles (1835–1873), Richard Colles (1844–1929) and the writer, have failed to identify this William Colles, owing to the absence of some key parish registers for that period, and also the loss of the early history of the family in a house fire in Dublin in a later century. John A. Purefoy Colles believed that William Colles, the progenitor of the Irish branch of the family, was one of the seven sons of William Colles (1560–1615) of Leigh, who are depicted in the Leigh church monument and three of whom are not recorded in the British Museum pedigree, which was based on the Herald's visitation of 1619, at which time one of the sons was already established in Ireland. Richard Colles, after extensive but inconclusive correspondence with the College of Arms, thought that his English ancestor was a son of Michael Colles of Hampton-in-Arden, the second son of William Colles the elder, of Leigh (1495–1558). Another suggestion is that this missing ancestor may have been the son of Edmund Colles (b. 1566) of Grimley, Worcestershire. Finally, the writer located a William Colles of Lulsley who died in 1596, and there is a document in the Worcester archives granting powers of administration of his estate to his widow, Margaret Colles, and to William Coles (?). We do not know whether this William Colles of Lulsley had a family, as the parish registers do not cover that period. It does however, prove that there were other members of the family of Colles of Leigh in the neighbourhood in the late sixteenth century. Further historical research will no doubt identify this Elizabethan youth, William Colles by name, who was to seek his fortune in Ireland.

The Irish branch of the Colles family springs from this William Colles of Doughill (1585–1621) (see Appendix)—who arrived in Ireland in the closing years of Elizabeth's reign. He was on the staff of a John Harrington, who we know came from the Coventry area. The age group of young Colles suggests that he was a page or courier, not an uncommon post for an impecunious but intelligent youth in the household of the nobility of that age. Harrington was secretary to the Earl of Essex and was knighted by him in Ireland. Essex preferred negotiation instead of fighting the great Irish leader, O'Neill, and incurred the Queen's displeasure and later the loss of his head. Harrington suffered only Her Majesty's displeasure at acceptance of his knighthood, but fortunately kept his head. The young Colles, now a soldier of fortune, in that Age of Conquest, acquired land and property at Doughill, County Roscommon, near the city of Athlone, then an important outpost for the new colonists. William Colles returned to England to engage eight gentlemen and thirty yeoman from Coleshill and Caldecote, North Warwickshire, and from Drayton in Leicestershire, to accompany him to Ireland and settle in his extensive estates. He also contacted his uncle, Rodger Purefoy. This Purefoy cannot be identified, although we do know that the Colles and Purefoy families were united by marriage in the reign of Henry VI and that the family also settled in Ireland. We know little of William Colles of Doughill, other than that "he died young, aged 36, in the year 1621 after encountering a variety of fortune". He married, and the careers of his three sons illustrate the turbulence of that age.

1. Job Colles was born in 1607, served as a soldier under King Gustavus of Sweden, the great champion of Protestantism, and was wounded in the Battle of Leipzig in 1631; dying from wounds received there some twenty years later. Gustavus presented him with a sword, which was in the possession of the Colles family a century later. Job Colles wrote a history of his ancestors, which was the one that was unfortunately lost in the family house fire later. Apparently in this history he described the ghost of old Colles (Edmund Colles, the younger) who rode his chariot through Leigh Manor.

2. William Colles, the second son, was born in 1610. He settled in Skinners Row, now Christchurch Place, Dublin, and carried on a successful business as an optician. He lost his

wife and two children in the Irish Rebellion of 1641, and escaping to Coventry, remarried there. Some years later he returned to Dublin and resumed his business. By his second marriage William had five sons and a daughter, some of whom were born in England. The eldest son Christopher became a clergyman in Derbyshire, and the second son William qualified as a surgeon to settle eventually in Kilkenny (vide infra). It was most probably one of the other sons, Charles (b. 1651), John (b. 1654) or Adrian (b. 1657) who published an important diary of events in Ireland during the William III–James II war (1685–1690); which concludes with a description of the entry into Dublin of the army of William after the Boyne victory. "God blessed us with a sight of many of our absent friends, but more abundantly with the never to be forgotten sight of glorious King William. There was great joy, and sorrow and sadness was gone away when we crept out of our houses and found ourselves in a new world. . . . Here endeth the tyranny, oppression, arbitrary power, will and pleasure, against all law, all charity and Christianity, all promises, and assurances made by a Popish Prince to a most dutiful people, the Protestants of Dublin."

3. Charles Colles, the third son, was born in 1616. He was a captain in the Royalist army in Ireland, but later switched his allegiance to the forces of Cromwell, which action his descendants are not very proud of. However, Charles benefited considerably, receiving large grants of lands in Sligo, Wexford and Kilkenny, in all some 2296 Irish acres. He was Provost Marshal of Connaught and later High Sheriff of Co. Sligo. He had a difficult job in a dangerous age and many stories, perhaps all apocryphal, are associated with his career. He was stated to have a gallows erected near his home, Collesford, near Magheramore in Co. Sligo, so that sentences could be expedited. Surprisingly he died in bed in the year 1685. His funeral entry in the Ulster King-at-Arms office in Dublin Castle bears the arms and crest of Colles of Leigh.

In the third generation, we continue with William Colles of Kilcollen (1648–1719). He was the second son of William Colles of Christchurch Place, Dublin and was born in England during his father's temporary sojourn there. He became an eminent surgeon in Kilkenny. At first he decided to follow his uncle Job's profession and become a soldier of fortune, later he decided on the ministry, but abandoned the idea on account of a speech impediment and chose chirurgery, which "demand the head and the hand rather than the tongue". He was sent to Coventry to school, and later as an apprentice he studied physic and chirurgery under the celebrated Lodge of Greenwich. In 1671 he went as a ship's surgeon to Lisbon, then more study in London followed, and finally, he went back to complete his education with Lodge until 1674. When qualified he appears to have been flitting about from Coventry to Sheffield and had to flee the latter city on account of a love affair, to settle finally in Kilkenny. He was apparently a very successful surgeon and became an important person locally. He purchased from the Kilkenny Corporation large estates of confiscated properties including the townlands of Kilcollen, Maudleen and Lisna-fulshin through his friendship with James, 2nd Duke of Ormonde. His first wife died childless, but with two subsequent wives he was father of fourteen children of whom five died young. In family circles he is referred to as "Brown Billy" on account of the colour of his portraits, of which there were many—he had one painted every seven years "to remind him of the lapse of life". It is stated that his great grandson Abraham Colles, while gazing at one of these portraits at Millmount, determined him to become a surgeon. At one time this William Colles was abducted from his home, imprisoned and tortured for three days in the caves at Dunmore—a deed attributed rightly or wrongly to the Papists. His great estates and fortunes passed to his eldest son, Barry, a barrister, who was twice Mayor of Kilkenny, but as this son, Barry, had no male heir, they passed on at the marriage of his daughter, Susanna, to the Meredyth family.

William Colles of Abbeyvale (1702–1770) was the second son of the surgeon and like many a second son had a difficult start in life. Being of a large family he was brought up by his aunt Elizabeth Colles who had lost her only child. Elizabeth was possessed of singular beauty and married three wealthy hus-bands. She, however, lost all in love and litigation and died penniless; her young nephew had to pay her funeral expenses.

William's father having died previously, and assumed that his
son was well provided for, left him only £100 in his will, and
also his proud uncle's tarnished sword. He was fortunately,
however, well qualified to make his own way, being a man
of untiring energy and universal talent, besides being endowed
with superior education and pre-eminent as a mathematician
and a mechanician. In early life he had also some pretensions
as a poet and wrote several tragedies. He acquired the lease of
the marble quarry, which was previously worked by hand. He
invented machinery for cutting, boring and polishing marble,
and built an industry which for close on two centuries made the
city of Kilkenny famous by giving it a valuable export product.
He had a scheme for supplying the corporation of Dublin with
bored marble tubes for water mains, but a combination of
pump borers and other mechanics rose in a mob and destroyed
them on their arrival in the city. English visitors in 1748 were
amazed at the massive blocks of marble that were quarried and
conveyed to the mill by mechanical contrivances of his invention. They saw warehouses attached to this mill filled with
marble products—chimney pieces, cisterns, buckets, vases,
punch bowls, mugs, frames for looking-glasses and pictures,
"that would employ the eye the longest day and yet find something to admire". No one could imitate this machinery—it
was perpetually at work night and day and required little
attention. He was, to use the words of another, a man of great
mechanical abilities and abounding in a variety of eccentric
schemes such as mark original genius, one of which was an
attempt to make dogs weave linen by turning wheels. While he
amused the populace by various devices, such as that of a
musical instrument resembling an Aeolian harp which played
by itself as it floated on the stream of the river, and many others,
he applied himself as well to the construction of useful machinery
for different purposes, inventing among other things a cider mill,
a water engine, and an engine for dressing flax, simple and
efficacious, though now superseded. Such was the impression
that his abilities made on the common people, that his feats
were proverbial among them and they spoke of him as a
necromancer. Some good examples of his marble products now
adorn St. Canice's Cathedral, Kilkenny. Like his brother,

Barry, he was twice Mayor of that city, and much of his correspondence survives. He was, for example, often addressing
himself to the growing problem of mendicity in Ireland and
suggested that the large beggar population should be taught a
trade, such as spinning. He advocated a canal linking the Nore
and Barrow rivers, which was only partially completed. Even
that famous sword did not escape the attention of that restless
genius. He had its hilt fashioned into a pair of buckles with an
inscription verse on them and later his son had these converted
into two small goblets and a snuff box. This William Colles lived
in those great early decades of the eighteenth century, which
were for many and different reasons a comparatively peaceful
era in Irish history, but this Age of Reason, this Augustan Age,
was soon to disappear forever in the tragic cataclysms at home
and abroad. William Colles, this great citizen of Kilkenny,
died in 1770 and there remains today a fine monument on the
exterior of St. Mary's Church, Kilkenny, inscribed—

"To the memory of Alderman William Colles, whose steady
attention to all religious and civic duties gained him the love
of his fellow citizens and whose ingenuity procured him the
admiration of strangers. By an uncommon genius he discovered and by an unwearying application and patience the
art of sawing, boring and polishing marble by water mill,
which by lowering the price of that valuable manufacture,
rendered its use more extensive. His whole life was employed
in works beneficial to society. His manner was inoffensive,
and his conduct always upright. He died on the 8th of March
1770 in the 68th year of his age.
"This monument was erected by his afflicted son William in
testimony of his reverence for the memory of so excellent a
father."

The inscription is prefaced by "Inventas aut qui vitam excoluere
per artis".* Virgil's next line—"Quique sui memores alios
fecere merendo", would also be appropriate for William's
grandson Abraham Colles. William Colles of Abbeyvale was
twice married, first to Sarah, widow of Lieutenant Robert

*Who enabled life by arts discovered.
  With all whose service to their kind won them remembrance among men.

Wheeler, by whom he had one daughter, and second to Rachel, widow of the Revd. Mathew Gibson, D.D., ex-Fellow of Trinity, by whom he had four sons.

William Colles of Millmount (1745–1779) son of the distinguished Kilkenny citizen and father of our subject, received his early education in the celebrated Quaker School at Ballitore in County Kildare, founded and carried on for many years by the Shackleton family—incidentally the ancestors of the famous explorer. Edmund Burke was educated at that school, and, though not contemporary with William, they did meet later, and William was a frequent visitor to the statesman's home in London. William was apparently unsettled in youth and tried to run away to sea, but was hauled back from Cork, and eventually settled down in the family marble business. He built himself Millmount House in 1770, a few miles from Kilkenny. This Georgian house still remains, although not now occupied by the Colles family. A year later, 1771, William married Mary Anne Bates, daughter of Abraham Bates of County Wexford, by whom he had three sons, William (b. 1772), Abraham (b. 1773), Richard (b. 1774), and a daughter, Rachel (b. 1776). William was never a robust individual, following an accident early in life, and died in 1779 at the early age of thirty-four. He was buried with the Quakers at Ballitore, for whom he retained the affection of his school days, and to whose tenets he had some year previously conformed; his wife and children remaining members of the Protestant Established Church of Ireland. His wife often teased him about his Quaker sympathies, and especially did not approve of the broad-brimmed hat which he and all Quaker men wore at the time. One day in a fit of petulance she took up a pair of scissors and trimmed the brim in a liberal manner. On taking up the hat to put it on, his sole remark was, "Oh, Mary, I see thou art minded to make a gamecock of me". His widow outlived him for more than sixty years, dying in the year 1840 at the age of ninety, and was buried at Maddoxtown, County Kilkenny.

CHAPTER 3

The Early Years

"One charge alone we give to youth:
Against the sceptred myth to hold
The golden heresy of Truth"

AE (G. W. Russell)

Abraham Colles, the second son of William Colles (1745–1779), was born in the family home, Millmount, Kilkenny, on the 23rd July 1773, his birth being announced to his uncle, Richard Colles of St. Stephen's Green, Dublin as follows:

23rd July, 1773

Dear Brother,

My dear Mary, at 3 o'clock this morning, made me the joyful father of a fine little thing—one of the light infantry.

William.

In subsequent letters his father mentioned that the child was christened Abraham after his maternal grandfather Abraham Bates, that "he was very small and neat", and that his smallness and delicacy occasioned his parents much anxiety. Nevertheless, this feeble infant became in due time a fairly tall, stout and strong man. When Abraham was five years old his father died, but this loss was largely compensated by the ability and devotion of his mother, a woman of superior intelligence and strongly imbued with religious principles. Colles was much attached to his mother and his devotion to her continued throughout her long life. He was sent, with his brothers, to the preparatory school of Mr. William Lindsay in Kilkenny, and the school fees for the term ending January 1783 were certainly very moderate, as the following account shows:

"To one quarter's boarding and schooling Master
Abraham Colles ending December 6th, 1782 —   £3. 8. 3d.

To one quarter's boarding and schooling Master
William Colles ending January 18th, 1783   —   £3. 8. 3d.

To one quarter's boarding and schooling Master
Richard Colles ending January 18th, 1783   —   £3. 8. 3d.

To paper for Master Abraham   —   £0. 0. 8d.
                                                  ──────────
                                                  £10. 5. 5d.

With his brothers, Abraham later entered Kilkenny College
under the Reverend John Ellison, headmaster. This famous
public school, one of the oldest in Ireland, was founded in 1538
by Piers, 8th Earl of Ormonde. It was closed for a time in the
next century owing to the political eclipse of the House of
Ormonde and the religious unrest at the time. After the
Restoration there was a change in the fortunes of the Ormonde
family, and James, now 1st Duke of Ormonde, re-established
and re-sited the College on the banks of the Nore in 1668,
where it still flourishes after three centuries. It was referred to
as the "Eton of Ireland" on account of the sons of the nobility
who were educated there, especially in the eighteenth century;
but there were even greater names than these on the Kilkenny
College roll; no other school in these islands has produced a
trio to compare with Berkeley, Swift and Congreve;   and
Wellington's generals, Pack, Cole, Pakenham and Beresford
were nurtured on its playing fields.

Kilkenny—grey limestone city of Norman foundation, on
the banks of the Nore, has long been an important place. Its
many spires, sung by Spenser, are mindful of Oxford. It was
once the seat of an Irish Parliament. James II granted its
physicians a Royal Charter in 1689, but no more was heard
of this after that King's hurried departure in the following year.
Its magnificent Tolsel remains. Its mayor's sword recalls that
it was repaired when Barry Colles was its mayor, and St. John's
Bridge was built during the mayoralty of his brother William.
Colles was certainly a great name in a proud city, and is

appropriately commemorated by a marble plaque near the west door of the Cathedral of St. Canice:—

IN MEMORY OF SOME MEMBERS OF THE FAMILY OF COLLES
FORMERLY OF LEIGH, CO. WORCESTER,
WHO WERE CONNECTED WITH KILKENNY.

CHARLES COLLES	of Magheramore, Co. Sligo, and Rahealy, Co. Kilkenny, H.S., Co. Sligo, 1685. Buried in the Chancel of St. Michael's Church, Dublin.
WILLIAM COLLES	of Kilcollen and Madeleen, Co. Kilkenny, died 1719. Buried in the Family Vault, St. Mary's Church, Kilkenny.
BARRY COLLES	of Kilcollen, and of St. Stephen's Green, Dublin, died 1785. Buried in Meredyth Vault, St. Patrick's Cathedral, Dublin.
WILLIAM COLLES	of Abbeyvale, and Patrick Street, Kilkenny, died 1770. Buried in the Family Vault, St. Mary's Church, Kilkenny.
WILLIAM COLLES	of Millmount, died 1779. Buried in Quaker Cemetery, Ballitore, Co. Kildare.
RICHARD COLLES	of Prospect, Co. Dublin and Parliament House, Kilkenny. Barrister-at-Law. Died 1815.
ABRAHAM COLLES	of Stephen's Green, Dublin, and Bonnettstown, Kilkenny. Died 1843, buried in Mount Jerome Cemetery, Dublin.
RICHARD COLLES	of Riverview, and of Ruthstown, Co. Kilkenny. Died 1849, buried at Maddockstown, Kilkenny.
ALEXANDER COLLES	of Millmount, died 1876, buried at Maddockstown, Kilkenny.
RICHARD COLLES	J.P. of Co. Kilkenny, died November 27th, 1929 at Kew, Surrey.

Colles had an excellent groundwork in the classics under Ellison, that famous headmaster. In September, 1790 he entered Trinity College, Dublin with his brother, William, and in the

same month was indentured to Philip Woodroffe, surgeon to
Dr. Steevens' Hospital. Colles had as tutor in Trinity the
Reverend Joseph Stopford, a genial and kindly man, and took
up residence there in December of that year. Colles was lucky
in his choice of tutor: had he been under the Reverend John
Walker, a fellow and tutor at that time, his story might have
been different. Walker was very unorthodox in his religious
beliefs and later resigned his fellowship to found an extreme
Calvinistic sect in Dublin. The "Walkerites", following the
teaching of St. Paul, greeted one another with a kiss, which
naturally led to confusion and ribaldry in practice. The movement later faded out in splinter groups of "Osculists" and "Non-
Osculists". Walker was later employed as a private tutor to
the great William Stokes.

John Hely-Hutchinson was then Provost of the College. He
was an undistinguished graduate of the University; later he
became a barrister and member of Parliament, and finally
Secretary of State in the Irish Parliament. By political intrigue
he secured this important post, and with no academic experience he was continually at loggerheads with his fellows.
Enlarging the Provost's House to accommodate his large
family and their many servants, he banished the Muses from
the Fellows' garden. Horse-riding, fencing, dancing, and
duelling in the student body, and the establishment of chairs in
modern languages, then a startling innovation, were in his view
more befitting preparations for the Grand Tour. Hely-
Hutchinson, generally referred to as "the Prancer" was the
subject of scurrilous publications, which had such an effect
on the public mind that an official letter expressing the King's
approval of his conduct as Provost was necessary. But when all
this is said, Hely-Hutchinson emerges as one of the great
Provosts of the eighteenth century. He was a strong advocate of
Catholic emancipation and regarded as disgraceful the restrictions imposed on Catholics in the University by requiring them
to take obnoxious oaths before admission to degrees. The year
before his death in 1794 such religious tests were abolished,
although certain restrictions on fellowships and scholarships
remained and were gradually removed in the following century.
But perhaps the most extraordinary character in Trinity in

those days was "Jacky" Barrett, fellow, bursar, and later
Vice-Provost, who was probably the most eccentric don ever
produced in the academic world. Barrett, learned in all
subjects, was able to converse fluently "in any language other
than his own". Also in that year, 1790, Edmund Burke received
an honorary LL.D. from his old Alma Mater, and in expressing
thanks for it stated that "the University was highly generous
in accepting with so much indulgence the produce of its own
gifts". The Historical Club founded by Burke in his student
days in 1747 was now continued as the College Historical
Society, and was the great centre of College student life; both
Abraham and his brother William were members. Practically
all the great figures in the Irish Parliament and the professions
received their early training in its debating halls, and its large
membership of over 800 suggests that graduates, ex-students,
and others, were all eligible; as in 1792 there were only 933
undergraduates in the University. It is now impossible to
determine, in the absence of initials, which of the Colles
brothers took part in the debates, became officers of the
Society, and received its medals. Abraham's brilliant per-
formances at the Speculative Society of Edinburgh years later
certainly suggests that he was already an experienced and
polished performer. The closing decades of the eighteenth
century provided varied and exciting subjects for debate.
England was in a desperate plight after the loss of the American
colonies, her King was mad, and there was a Regency crisis.
There were repercussions of the French Revolution, now at its
height, and finally the great war with France in 1793. At home,
after a peace of 100 years, Ireland now demanded its freedom
and the emancipation of its Catholic population. Societies of
United Irishmen, originally founded in Belfast by Wolfe Tone,
a Protestant, and a student of Trinity, now mushroomed
through the land. Trinity in those days contained several cells
of United Irishmen and naturally the College Historical Society
debates became more political. After several warnings from the
College authorities and attempts by them to control its activities, the Society abandoned their college rooms in 1794 and
took up quarters in the city. Abraham Colles was a member of
this "Extern" Society in 1795. This, then, is the background of

Colles in Trinity. He was an arts student only; though he attended two courses of lectures in the medical school there, under Robert Perceval (chemistry) and Stephen Dickson (practice of medicine), he did not matriculate in that school. The reasons for this will be given later. His brother William did brilliantly in his arts course, becoming a scholar of the house and a prizeman of the University, but left Trinity without a degree. Possibly, like many others at that time, he was not in sympathy with his Alma Mater.

On arrival in Dublin in that year 1790, as a young lad of seventeen, Colles was already decided on a surgical career. His great grandfather, whose portrait was at Millmount, may have been his boyhood hero. There is another story, that he picked up a textbook of anatomy floating in the Nore after the flooding of a neighbour's house. The doctor owner presented Abraham with it and the youth read it carefully. Colles was proof from the first against every seduction that sought to win him from the profession of his choice. He embraced it with the ardour of a lover and paid it no divided allegiance. An anecdote connecting his name with that of Edmund Burke ought not to be omitted. His uncle, Richard Colles, at whose house he was now a frequent visitor, had some dispute with a London bookseller concerning the publication and copyright of a satirical poem; and he had a correspondence with Mr. Burke upon the subject. Mr. Burke's letter suggested to the young student some remarks "on the conditions of political satire" which he hastily committed to paper and showed to his uncle, who privately sent them to his illustrious acquaintance in England. Mr. Burke returned them with encomiums on their spirit and good sense, even recommending their publication. The author, however, when desired by his gratified relative to prepare them for the press, thrust the papers into the fire, and, when his uncle talked of the "name" which he was sacrificing, replied, "A name, Sir! Yes, as an author; and then not a dowager in Dublin would call me in to cure a sore throat."

A few weeks after entry into Trinity, Colles was indentured to Philip Woodroffe of Dr. Steevens' Hospital and became a registered pupil of the Surgeons' School of the Royal College of Surgeons in Ireland. Apprenticeship was then the standard system of surgical training. The system raised the prestige of the master as well as being lucrative. Minimum fees were £200 if resident, or £100 if non-resident, but fees of £300–£500 were not uncommon in those days. The apprenticeship system was compulsory for the Royal College of Surgeons in Ireland diploma until 1825, when it became optional and was dispensed with under their new charter of 1844. It was a system open to abuse by unscrupulous masters, and the Irish College limited apprentices to two for each member and the members required the council's permission to take on any extra pupils. At that time there were between twenty and thirty apprentices in Dr. Steevens' Hospital. For these youths life was an arduous calling, as they had ever to be at their master's call and mercy. Badly housed in any old corner of the hospital, poorly fed, these tender youths had to hold down struggling patients on the operating tables of those pre-anaesthetic days, handing their masters the knives and other instruments of the trade, and taking hold of the amputated limbs. They had to work in the overcrowded wards and attempt to calm terror-stricken and dying patients; all this in the presence of blood—fresh and stale, pus, and the stench of gangrene. In those pre-Listerian days all patients' wounds went septic, and the flow of pus was so commonplace that it was referred to as "good", "healthy", "laudable" or otherwise. The pain and misery of these wretched patients left their mark on young Colles, and his afterwork had the hallmark of compassion, especially for the sick poor.

That bold band of Dublin surgeons who received their Royal Charter in 1784 were without funds, prospects or patronage. Lacking in everything except courage, their enthusiasm and vigour infected, inspired, and fascinated youth. Under their charter they established a medical school and appointed as professors: Dease (surgery); Hallahan and Hartigan (anatomy and physiology); Hallahan (midwifery); and Archer (surgical pharmacy). Looking around for a suitable building, they acquired a ramshackle house at the back of Mercer's Hospital in 1789 which they renovated, but for which they were not able to pay the contractors for some years. The ground floor was converted into a dissecting room, with a few tables and pinewood forms arranged in a semi-circle. A room upstairs was the council room, examination room, and library combined. In the following year, 1790, young Colles entered this School as a registered pupil and his admission cards to lectures and dissections for the years 1790–1793 still survive. In that year also, John Hunter was made an honorary member of the Royal College of Surgeons in Ireland and presented the College with copies of his books. The number of students attending the first sessions are not available, but in 1792 there were 100 students, most of whom were destined for the armies of Pitt. We will now take leave of Colles in the dissecting room and lecture halls of the Surgeons' School, attending his master at Dr. Steevens' Hospital and his arts course at Trinity. He also attended the House of Industry* for one winter session. He will emerge five years later as an arts graduate (B.A.) of the University and a licentiate or holder of "Letters Testimonial" of the Royal College of Surgeons in Ireland. Meanwhile, we will take a quick look at other parts of the Irish medical scene, the University and the Physicians, which fortunately are inter-related.

Ireland's oldest and greatest seat of learning, the University of Dublin, usually referred to by the name of its single College—Trinity College, Dublin—was founded by Queen Elizabeth in 1591. The reader will no doubt like to be reminded that this was the Alma Mater of Berkeley, Swift, Goldsmith and Burke. By its means that monarch hoped "to subdue the turbulence and barbarism of the Irish, to introduce civility, and to make it unnecessary for its natives to travel to France, Italy and Spain, to get learning in such foreign universities, whereby they have been infected with Popery and all ill qualities, and so become evil subjects". This was the language of the Age of Conquest, but in spite of its terms the University survived, although the political upheavals, wars, and rebellions in the succeeding century were not conducive to its development and to the cultivation of learning. Yet the great English historian, G. M. Trevelyan, was later to write:

> "A unique institution, which for three and a half centuries has embraced so much of what was best, greatest and happiest

* Later named The Richmond Hospital, now St. Laurence's Hospital.

in the chequered career of Ireland. The proportion of famous Irish names upon its rolls is wonderful—names of poets, satirists, novelists, orators, scientists, historians, men of learning in every branch of study, publicists and politicians of every party. What other College, I had almost said what other University, could show a nobler roll? [One is struck by] the liberality of Trinity College in days when little else in Ireland was liberal. Furthermore, in the eighteenth century, when almost all the other established and endowed institutions in the British Isles were struck with paralysis, when Oxford and Cambridge declined shamefully in numbers, in enterprise and in reputation, the Alma Mater of Edmund Burke was flourishing and adorning herself with new buildings. The character and achievement of Trinity, Dublin, has been due to Irishmen."

Unfortunately this historian's encomiums could not always have been bestowed on the Trinity medical school. At its foundation in 1591 the University intended to establish a faculty of medicine and grant degrees, but no regulations for these were established until about 1620, and only one medical degree was conferred in the first twenty-three years of its existence. We find in 1628 an apologetic letter from Provost Bedell to Archbishop Ussher—"I suppose it has been an error all this while to neglect the faculties of law and physic and attend only to the ordering of one poor College of divines". In 1626 Charles I advocated a College of Physicians in Dublin similar to the London College, but the Irish Rebellion of 1641, the English civil war and the commonwealth intervened. Meanwhile John Stearne, a scholar of Trinity, had to flee Ireland during the Rebellion and studied at Cambridge and Oxford, returning in 1654 to a fellowship in Trinity and a professorship of Hebrew four years later. In 1660 he was appointed president of a fraternity of Physicians at Trinity Hall. Trinity Hall, originally intended as the Bridewell of the city but never used as such, was sold to Trinity as a hostel for its students; it was at the west end of Hoggen Green (now College Green) and outside the city walls. Stearne was also elected professor of medicine in the University. In 1667 he obtained a charter for the College

of Physicians from Charles II. Under this arrangement the
University and the Physicians were integrated and worked in
harmony for some twenty years.

Now we are at war again. William of Orange and James II
were destined to fight it out in Ireland, and that battle, in
addition to other consequences, brought forth a medical figure
who, for personality, a celebrated will, and the machinations
that led to the establishment of a hospital bearing his name,
could well provide ample material for an Abbey Theatre play.
Patrick Dun was born at Aberdeen in 1642 and graduated
there and also at Oxford and at continental universities. He
came to Ireland, became a fellow and later president of the
College of Physicians, and physician to the Army, presumably
that of James II. He left Ireland, and we next find him with
William's army on the Boyne. William was apparently shot at
by a trigger-happy sentry the night before the battle, and his
surgeons considered it unwise that he should be present; Dun
however disagreed and pronounced the monarch fit for duty.
In 1692 Dun obtained a new charter for the Physicians' College
from William and Mary and was once more elected president
of the College. He fought a celebrated duel with Dr. Howard
in York Street in 1693, which was the subject of numerous
ballads.

> "As for the motives most men doubt
> Why these two doctors did fall out,
> Some say it was ambition
> and that one did undermine
> The other's credit, with design
> To be the State Physician."

Patrick Dun was now all powerful and had acquired a knighthood (1696), a large practice, wealth, and vast estates. As
early as 1704 he intimated that in his will he would establish
a professorship of medicine in Dublin under the Physicians'
control. This stimulated the University to establish their own
medical school, "which was opened with due ceremony and
recitation of verses" in 1711—a two-storied building at the
south-east corner of the library, and shown in eighteenth-
century prints of the College. This little medical school had

lectureships in anatomy, surgery, botany, chemistry, natural philosophy, and medicine. Dun died in 1713 and his celebrated will dated 1711 was the subject of court actions and Acts of Parliament for two-and-a-half centuries. He left the life interest of his estates, then about £6,000, to Lady Dun as long as she remained a widow, which condition naturally upset her, and even Archbishop King's soothing diplomacy—"I am sure he loved you with a cordial and conjugal affection, and could not, with ease to himself, think of any others enjoying you"—did not allay her wounded pride. Two years after Dun's death the professorship known as that of "The King's professor of Physic in the city of Dublin" was established by Royal Charter, but the first two occupants of its chair did not lecture, as there was no salary—Lady Dun being still alive. Various court actions were necessary to get them a salary and this was not possible until 1749, when three King's professors, Quin, Barry and Barbor, were appointed at £100 each per annum, and this rose gradually to over £300 per annum. There were apparently no duties attached, and there is no record of any one of these giving any lectures; they simply enjoyed this professorial sinecure for 42 years, 36 years and 34 years respectively. In a poem descriptive of the Medical Faculty in Dublin, published by John Gilborne, M.D., in 1775, the following lines are devoted to the King's Professors—

Peculiar Laurels the next Three have won,
Professors Royal of *Sir Patrick Dun*;
A good Physician and a worthy Knight,
To cure not kill was always his delight.
If any Time he drew the trenchant Blade,
The Hand that wounded heal'd the Wounds it made.

Ingenious *Quin*, with Erudition great,
Averts the Blows of unrelenting Fate:
He teaches Youth the Cure, the Remedies,
And various Causes of all Maladies;
And the best Practice in the Physic-school.

The God-like *Barry* high in Learning soars,
His prudent Skill the Sick to Health restores:
He teaches Midwifes how to trace their Clews

Thro' mazy Labyrinths, and how to use
Their Instruments he shews Chirurgeons bold;
All this in College by the Sage is told.

Wise *Barbor* can prolong the Days of Youth,
By Maxims founded on undoubted Truth:
With pharmaceutic Art he plainly shews
How to prepare, preserve, compound, and chuse
Drugs, and Materials medical, that will
All Indications curative fulfil.

It is said that von Haller, Albinus and Van Swieten were willing
to compete for Dun's endowment if it had not been subdivided.
Had any of these great men been induced to make Dublin his
home, the medical school might in the eighteenth century have
become a rival to Leiden and Edinburgh.

Meanwhile, the University and the Physicians appeared to
be in harmony, the University producing its four or five
graduates annually, and the Physicians in practice acting as
examiners for these degrees, and later licensing those to practise
in the city of Dublin whom they, the Physicians, then limited
to fourteen fellows, considered themselves alone to control.
But all this was to end abruptly about 1760, in what came to be
known as the Ould imbroglio. Fielding Ould was then a leading
obstetrician in Dublin and attended Lady Mornington at the
birth of the future Duke of Wellington. He was the author of a
famous textbook of midwifery, and was later to be successor to
Bartholomew Mosse, as Master of The Lying-In Hospital
(Rotunda). He decided to take a medical degree, and fulfilled
the University requirements, as he was already a graduate in
arts. The Physicians, however, refused to examine him, and
considered themselves "treated with very great and undeserved
disrespect for being asked to do so", as their bye-laws did not
allow a physician to practise the undignified art of midwifery
at the same time. The Physicians' bye-laws do not, however,
appear to be consistent, as they were themselves granting licences to practice midwifery and Ould himself already had this
licence. The University then appointed their own examiners
and granted Ould his batchelor degree in medicine. The
Physicians then withdrew, and all contracts between the

University and the Physicians were now considered to have ended. Fielding Ould was later knighted, which honour gave rise to the following epigram:

> "Sir Fielding Ould is made a Knight
> He should have been a Lord by right:
> For then each Lady's prayer would be,
> O Lord, Good Lord, deliver me!"

One is happy to record that the Physicians repented and granted Ould their licence to practise medicine, a quarter of a century later.

The immediate result of the Ould imbroglio, and as it turned out for Trinity a happy one, was the resignation of Robert Robinson, then president of the College of Physicians, from the lectureship of anatomy and surgery at the University, and his replacement by George Cleghorn. Robinson was responsible for procuring the famous skeleton of Cornelius Magrath, which is now in the School of Anatomy at Trinity. Magrath suffered from gigantism and acromegaly and was 7 feet 8 inches high, with hands "as large as a middling shoulder of mutton". He exhibited himself as a giant in various cities in Ireland and abroad, and naturally his death was looked forward to by anatomists! When Magrath died, aged 24, Robinson addressed his class as follows: "Gentlemen, I have been told that some of you in your zeal have contemplated the carrying off of the body. I most earnestly beg of you not to think of such a thing, but if you should be carried away with your desire for knowledge, and thus against my expressed wish you persist in doing so, I would have you remember that if you take up the body there is no law whereby you can be touched, but if you take as much as a rag or a stocking with it, it is a hanging matter." The students took the hint and attended the wake of the giant, and as the evening progressed, drugged the whiskey used in the celebrations; when the friends gradually dropped off to sleep the students took the body unmolested to the College. Next morning the friends came with indignant protests to the Provost and demanded the return of the corpse. The Provost sent for Robinson, who assured him that so great was the diligence of the College students that the body was already dissected. Robinson, on his way back from the Provost, was stopping at intervals and chuckling to himself—"Divil a knife's in him yet!!", while the Provost was left to deal with the angry friends!

With the eclipse of Robinson, George Cleghorn, the University Anatomist, succeeded to the lectureship of anatomy and chirurgery. He was the best known figure in the Trinity medical school, which he served with distinction for some 36 years. Of farming stock, he was born in Cramond, near Edinburgh, in 1716. As a medical student in Edinburgh he came under the influence of Alexander Monro *Primus*, actually living in his home, and with four other students founded a medical society which emerged later as the Royal Medical Society of Edinburgh. After qualifying he entered the Army as a regimental surgeon, and while his regiment was stationed in Minorca he published a work *on the epidemic diseases of Minorca 1744–1749*, which went to five editions. He later studied under Hunter in London and on going to Ireland with his regiment he decided to stay in Dublin and practise as a surgeon. Elected University Anatomist in 1753, he published three years later *An Index of an Annual Course of Lectures*. Although essentially a syllabus this gives us a standard of the anatomical and surgical teaching available at that time. In 1762 he sent a paper to the Medical Society of London, in which he describes how he extracted "the third or fourth feather of a goose's wing" from the throat of a young lady who swallowed it. The instrument he used was a flexible whalebone with a spring and strings attached to it. In 1765 he described to the same Society a case of aneurysmal varix in the arm of a boy aged seventeen, which had resulted from a bleeding some years before—probably the first record of this lesion. In a small room in that small building some 90 students attended Cleghorn's lectures and demonstrations. His retirement in 1785 and death four years later was a great loss to the University and the chief factor in the decline of the school at that period. Cleghorn's fine character is illustrated in his reply to a junior soliciting his support for a medical appointment:

"My stomach revolts against the usual mode of extracting promises and engaging votes before the governors can be sufficiently apprized of the merits of the candidates. It is founded on the supposition that all men are actuated by selfish motives, regardless of the public good, and they never consider whether their friend be fit for the place he wishes for, provided the place be fit for him. If you gain the election I hope it will be by means fair and honourable; I would rather hear you had lost it, than that any others had been employed. The more a good character is enquired into, it will be so much the better for him who owns it; you must therefore be the gainer by standing the election, even should you fail of success, provided you are not too anxious about the matter, and suffer your mind to be too much dejected by a disappointment, which could not have happened had merit been regarded, and which, after all, may probably tend more to your advantage than success would have done. Read the tenth satire of Juvenal, and reflect on the vanity of human fears and wishes."

In a newspaper obituary (1789) Cleghorn is described as "a gentleman where ever known esteemed and beloved, and where ever heard of respected. For a series of years supporting with singular honour one of the most distinguished characters in his profession, he was the first person that established what could with any degree of propriety be called a school of anatomy in this Kingdom; which long flourished with still increasing splendour and utility under his auspices and direction and remains a lasting monument of his industry, spirit, and genius."

The grant of a Royal Charter to the Royal College of Surgeons in Ireland in 1784 and the declared intention of that body to establish its own medical school, stimulated the University and the Physicians to come together again. The School of Physic Act of 1785 established chairs of anatomy and surgery, botany, chemistry, and physic in the University. The Physicians nominated three King's professorships in the practice of medicine, the institutions of medicine, and materia medica and pharmacy. Of the six occupants of these original chairs, five were Edinburgh University M.Ds. The effect of this Act, however, was the opposite of what was expected, and in the last fifteen years of the eighteenth century the medical school reached almost the lowest level in its history. The establishment of clinical lectures proved an obstacle which the united wisdom of the Colleges was unable to overcome and the effort to solve this difficulty resulted in open rupture amongst the professors. The chief stars in the drama were Hill, Perceval and Dickson. Had Abraham Colles matriculated as a Trinity medical student in 1790 he would have been the only student doing so.

Among Abraham Colles's contemporaries in Trinity was young Robert Emmet, son of Dr. Robert Emmet, State Physician, and later to be hanged for his abortive rebellion in 1803. Thomas Moore was another fellow-student, and one of the first Roman Catholics to be free to take his degree without subscribing to abnoxious oaths. Moore was very attached to Emmet and the latter's love for Sarah Curran was the inspiration of several of his melodies.

Crossing the street from the great west front of Trinity (1760) Colles would enter Parliament House, his undergraduate gown serving as his admission ticket to its gallery. There he could enjoy the rich oratory of Grattan and Flood, and perhaps witness the political manoeuvres, bribery and corruption of the Fitzgibbon, Beresford and Castlereagh clique who a few years later were to sell that Irish Parliament as well as their honour. But even that tragic forum had its light relief. Witness the address of Sir Boyle Roche, member for Tralee and Master of Ceremonies at the Castle: "It would surely be better, Mr. Speaker, to give up not only a *part*, but if necessary, the *whole* of our constitution, to preserve the *remainder*", and again, "Why should we do anything for posterity? What has posterity ever done for us?". The latter philosophy has never lacked adherents in Ireland, but in spite of it, that generation, for all its faults, built a Georgian city we still rejoice in, and a series of majestic buildings which Macauley reminds us would not be out of place in the French capital. The Irish Parliament, still regarded by England's Treasury as representing mere colonists, to be taxed with their kind in Boston and New York, was only too happy to cut the profits of the London tax gatherers and to build for its people a comfortable capital.

In nearby Dublin Castle, Colles would have witnessed the pageantry, splendour and entertainment of that famous

Viceregal Court, second only in magnificence to that of London. Had he penetrated its great halls he would have noticed a young and gay army captain acting as A.D.C. to the Viceroy. This young soldier, Arthur Wellesley, born in Dublin, third son of Lord Mornington, the professor of music at Trinity, was soon to join his brothers in India and distinguish himself in military command. Napoleon, who styled him the "Sepoy General", was later to regret his contemptuous remark. As Wellington and Prime Minister he lived to emancipate his fellow countrymen in 1829—although this was at least thirty years too late.

From Trinity, Colles would have strolled down to the river— the Anna livia plurabelle of later-day Joyce, to view the new Carlisle bridge now nearing completion. This, then the city's most easterly bridge, was now to link up Westmoreland Street with the great, wide Sackville Street extending northwards beyond. This famous street, one of the widest in Europe, originally designed as an open space, now contained the town houses of the aristocracy of the Ascendancy. William Dease, Ireland's first professor of surgery, lived there with scores of peers as his neighbours, the same street that Oliver Gogarty strolled down so gaily in our day. At the north end of Sackville Street was Bartholomew Mosse's Rotunda Hospital, the first hospital built in Europe for woman in her hour of travail. Looking eastward down the river, the great Custom House (1781–1791), "Gandon's Glory" was now nearing completion, and north of this was the Gardiner estate of Georgian streets and squares now losing popularity as the residential area of the city. A few years before, Lord Kildare (later Duke of Leinster) built his great town house on the south side of the city, in Molesworth Fields, and proudly boasted that Dublin would follow him there. This indeed Dublin did, and as the eighteenth century closed the Georgian city extended southwards, by the rapid development of the Fitzwilliam and Merrion estates. From the Carlisle bridge—rebuilt, widened and re-named O'Connell Bridge in the following century, Colles would have seen the erection of the massive Four Courts—Dublin's Inns of Court, also built by Gandon (1786–1796). While further west in the south bank he could see the clock tower of Dr. Steevens' Hospital—the

oldest voluntary hospital in the British Isles, which was to
be his professional home for some fifty years. This was the
Georgian Dublin whose creators believed in civilisation and the
humanities.

> "Water and rock by warriors wed
> Here with the landscape well accord.
> They built beyond Time's ambuscade,
> Builders and wielders of chisel and sword,
> So well they dealt with stone and stream,
> Eternity deals well with them."
>
> Oliver Gogarty.
>
> *Others to Adorn* 1938.

Colles received his arts degree (B.A.) from Trinity in April
1795, and on the 24th September of the same year he received
the licence or "Letters Testimonial" of the Royal College of
Surgeons in Ireland. Even before that date he was doing some
private practice from the hospital, and his financial difficulties
at that time are illustrated in the following letter:—

"To: Revd. John Foresythe,
          Betaghstown, Kilcock.

Dear Sir,

You will readily conceive how particularly circumstanced
and how perfectly devoid of other resources I must be when
I take the liberty of requesting that (if convenient) you will
be kind enough to favour me within the course of ten days
with any sum of money which you have proposed as a recompense for my attendance during your illness. Be assured,
Sir, that nothing but a disappointment in the only other
quarter from whence I could derive it and an absolute necessity of paying their fees to the College of Surgeons on the 5th
of next month could have forced me thus far to be trouble-
some, perhaps rude, to one I so highly esteem. Please give
my best respects to all the family at Betaghstown and believe
me to be
                              Yours truly,

Dr. Steevens' Hospital,   A. Colles.
August 26th, 1795."

In September, 1795 Colles set out for Edinburgh, and the hazards of a sea voyage of some twenty miles, taking three days, and costing £8 9s. 6d. are described in his first letter home—

Wednesday,

"Dear Mother,

Thank God that I can tell you I have arrived at the land of Scotland and am now arrived at a town called Stranraer, one stage from Port Patrick, where we arrived at 6 o'clock this morn: We put to sea from Donaghadee on Sunday Morn, but such a tossing and such an escape no set of poor devils ever had. As we are in a hurry posting off to Ayr I cannot at present tell you more, but you shall have a journal when I get to Edinburgh."

"Thy sons, Edina! social, kind,
With open arms, the stranger hail;
Their views enlarg'd, their lib'ral mind,
Above the narrow, rural vale."
Robert Burns.
Address to Edinburgh—1786

Edinburgh is a proud and honoured name in the world of medicine, with a tradition older than Flodden Field. James IV who perished there with his entire army in 1513 was the same king who in 1506 confirmed the grant of a Royal Charter to the Barber Surgeons of Edinburgh by the Town Council the previous year. In this charter of 1505 provision was made for human dissection, which Russell rightly regards as "the cradle of anatomy" in these islands. "Considering the state of science and of the opinion regarding the propriety of dissection of the human body at this time, it is a remarkable circumstance that the importance and the practice of dissection as the ground work of the healing art had been thus early and wisely recognised by the municipal authorities of Edinburgh" (Struthers). We must remember that in 1505 Andreas Vesalius, the father of modern anatomy, was not then born, and it was more than a century before Harvey discovered the circulation of the blood. In Paris, as late as 1551, Du Bois (Sylvius) was still worshipping

and defending Galen, and teaching anatomy from small fragments of dogs. After this auspicious start the Edinburgh
Barber-Surgeons remained silent for almost two hundred
years, and we can only infer that they availed themselves of the
privileges secured for them by the terms of their charter by
instructing themselves and their apprentices in the anatomical
art. The Barber-Surgeons' guild was the most senior and
respected of the city of Edinburgh guilds, and we hope they
enjoyed the special privilege—now unfortunately lapsed, of
distilling and marketing *uisge beatha** in that city. Nevertheless,
the fact remains that those two centuries saw the renaissance
of human anatomy and surgery on the Continent, under the
great names of Vesalius, Fallopius, Vidius, Sylvius, Columbus,
Eustachius, Varolius, Fabricus, Malpighi and Ruysch, and of
course not forgetting our own William Harvey.

In 1694, Alexander Monteith, at the instigation of Archibald
Pitcairn, established a school of anatomy in Edinburgh but
this school lapsed after three years, as Monteith was not acting
in concert with his fellow members of the Barber-Surgeons'
guild, who opened their own anatomical theatre in 1697.
In 1705 Robert Eliot was appointed professor of anatomy by
the Town Council, who then controlled the University or
"Town College" as it was then called, the Town Council
providing the title and a small salary of £15 per annum, and
the Barber-Surgeons providing the anatomical theatre. This
happy arrangement was continued with Eliot's successors,
Adam Drummond and John McGill. These latter two joint
professors of anatomy were replaced in 1720 by Alexander
Monro *Primus*, a remarkably able man who became the real
founder of the Edinburgh School. Monro arranged to have
four physicians—St. Clair, Rutherford, Plummer and Innes,
from the recently chartered Physicians' College (1681) to teach
medicine and chemistry in the Surgeons' theatre. In 1725
Monro was forced to abandon the Surgeons' theatre following
public reaction to "resurrectionist" activities, and to establish
himself in the University. Here he was joined the following
year by his four medical colleagues, now as full professors of the
university. Thus the Edinburgh medical school dates officially

* *Whisky*—to Sassenachs!

from 1726 and it is to be noted that all five of its original professors had all been students of Leiden under the great Boerhaave. Monro also determined to have a hospital for clinical teaching and a small infirmary of some six beds was opened in 1729. Later, with the co-operation of Provost Drummond, a new Royal Infirmary was built between 1738 and 1741. This was a remarkable achievement by the citizens of Edinburgh and it provided beds for 228 patients. In the operating theatre, under its great dome, there was accommodation for 200 students and it was there that the famous surgeons, Lizars, Fergusson, Liston, and Syme performed their operations. This theatre served Edinburgh until 1879 when the new Royal Infirmary was built. Monro practised surgery and was possessed of a good clinical judgement. He tells us that of the fifty cases of breast carcinoma which he extirpated, only four were free of disease after two years. He remarked also, "People are too hasty in in making conclusions: a single case or two has too often been the occasion of fixing a general rule for the cure of disease". Monro had a class roll of 57 when he began in 1720, which continued to increase, and reached about 160 when he retired in 1758. He was succeeded by his son, Alexander Monro *Secundus*, who was even a greater man. The rapid development of this great medical school was due to the remarkable co-operation between Town, University, Physicians and Barber-Surgeons—a condition simply unthinkable at that time in Paris, London or Dublin. When Abraham Colles arrived in Edinburgh in September 1795, its medical school was at the peak of its fame and was attracting students from every land—the Irish usually forming the largest single national contingent. Colles was particularly unfortunate after having viewed in Trinity a chaotic medical scene following the failure of its professors to agree. He was now to enter a medical school which at that particular time was notorious for a singularly pugnacious professoriate, who abused one another in a manner which for audacity if not for bitterness would be well-nigh impossible at the present day. In that last decade of the eighteenth century there was also an extraordinary amount of nepotism prevailing in Edinburgh, as may be judged from the fact that of the ten university appointments eight went to sons of previous professors of the university. In several of these cases the appointments later proved to be unsatisfactory.

Then presiding over the university medical school was the great figure of Alexander Monro *secundus* (of the foramen), whose name is familiar to every medical man. He had a class roll of over 300 students, and he later estimated that up to 1807 some 13,404 students passed through his department, but only a small proportion of these graduated from the university. It simply meant that at that time Monro was the best teacher and attracted the greatest number of students. Later it was the turn of the great teachers of the extra-mural schools when the university numbers declined. Monro, brilliant anatomist as he was, was also a practising physician, and true to the Leiden tradition, he regarded surgery as a minor part of the anatomy course. In 1776 the surgeons advocated separation of their subject and the establishment of a separate chair of surgery in the university. Monro countered this by having the title of his chair altered in the following year to a professorship of anatomy, medicine and surgery, and he succeeded in keeping the surgeons out of the university in his lifetime, but his son and successor, Alexander Monro *Tertius* failed to maintain that arrangement and had to agree to Turner's appointment to a separate chair of surgery in 1831. Meanwhile, a chair of clinical surgery was established in 1803 and confined to the Royal Infirmary, and the surgeons established a chair of surgery in their own College in 1804.

At that time it was stated that "nobody could have died contented without having consulted Benjamin Bell", then the leading surgeon in Edinburgh, and regarded as the first of its scientific surgeons. He was one of the first surgeons to receive honorary membership of the Irish College during the first year of its charter in 1784. His *System of Surgery* in six volumes (1783–1788) modelled on Heister's System, published nearly half a century before, was the first attempt in English to bring together the art of surgery in broad and orderly form. He was the first to emphasise the importance of seeking for some means of preventing or diminishing pain in surgical operations, and also referred to the dangers of too frequent changes of dressings, and the admission of air which tended to retard healing. In his treatise, "Gonorrhoea Virulenta and Lues Venera" (1793), he clearly demonstrated that the poisons of gonorrhoea and syphilis were essentially different—opinions which ran counter to those of Hunter. And his widsom continues—"The ends the surgeon has in view are in general attainable by very simple means—to divest the art of all the useless machinery with which it had become encumbered, which tends more to evince the ingenuity of its authors than to render the operations for which it was intended, more easily accomplished." Colles attended his clinical lectures and in his later work in Dublin made many kind references to his old teacher.

Colles' other teacher was John Bell, who was no relation of Benjamin Bell, with whom he agreed in nothing but the surname! This dogmatic and outstanding teacher has not always been treated fairly by later historians, but Struthers, who was closer to his time, regarded him as a "bold and dexterous operator, who combined all the qualities—natural and acquired —of a great surgeon, to an extraordinary degree. He was original and fearless, and a thorough anatomist, he had intellect, nerve, and also language, and was master alike of head and hand, and tongue and pen, and he was laborious as well as brilliant". All are agreed that he was a talented man, a classical scholar, an accomplished musician, and a skilful artist. He opened his school of anatomy and surgery in Surgeons' Square, where he lectured for the ten years 1786–1796, attracting students away from the university, and thereby antagonising the powerful combination of Monro and Gregory, who successfully had him excluded from the Royal Infirmary staff. He defended himself stoutly and vigorously against the violence of Gregory's attacks. John Bell's greatest success was that he taught surgical anatomy and must be regarded as one of its pioneers. There can be little doubt that it was he who stimulated young Colles' interest in that subject as the first publication of Colles was a treatise on surgical anatomy—a slim little volume, but the first of its kind. Bell stated that the surgeon should be as familiar with the anatomy of the parts as if he had made them. Bell's view, perhaps biased, in referring to Monro's class— "Unless there be a fortunate succession of bloody murders, not three subjects were dissected in a year. On the remains of a

subject fished up from the bottom of a tub of spirit, are demonstrated those delicate nerves which are to be avoided or divided
in our operations, and these are demonstrated once at a distance
of 100 ft.—nerves and arteries which the surgeon has to dissect
at the peril of the patient's life". Excluded from the Royal
Infirmary, John Bell also gave up his anatomy school to his
younger brother and assistant, Charles, and became the leading
surgeon of Edinburgh after the death of Benjamin Bell in 1806.
He died young, aged 57, while on a holiday to Rome in 1820,
and his grave lies next to that of John Keats. Young Charles
Bell, later the great Sir Charles Bell, was also contemporary
with Colles in Edinburgh. He was to continue his brother's
school, but like him was also forced out, by the same combination against his brother, to achieve fame in London. Edinburgh
made some amends by having him back in the chair of surgery
some thirty years later, but it was then too late for both. Two
other anatomists were students with Colles. Alexander Monro
Tertius graduated M.D. with him in 1797. Monro *Tertius* was
to succeed his father, but was not of the same calibre, and under
him the great anatomy school lost its lustre and its students to
the extra-mural school of John Barclay. John Barclay was 36
years old when he qualified in 1796, as he had previously been a
clergyman. It was typical of that peaceful and modest man that
he should dedicate his M.D. thesis to the great antagonists
John Bell and James Gregory! Barclay took over the school of
anatomy vacated by the brothers, John and Charles Bell, and
attracted some 300 students to his classes. He was the first
whole-time anatomist and never practised. The appointment
of Monro *Tertius* to the university chair has always been
criticised, as Edinburgh had then more able men available—
the brothers John and Charles Bell, and John Barclay.

Dominating Edinburgh medicine at that time was the
powerful figure of James Gregory. He had succeeded the great
Cullen in the chair of medicine in 1790. He was a most able
teacher, and increased his popularity still further by being the
leader in the professional controversies and the diverting
publications by which he used to maintain and enliven them.
His disposition towards personal attack was his besetting sin.
True to his character, Gregory's measures for the cure of disease

were sharp and incisive. There was no question of expectant treatment with him. Disease, according to Gregorian physic, was to be attacked vigorously by free blood-letting, the cold effusion, brisk purging, frequent blisters, and vomits of tartar emetic. Since Edinburgh, during his regime, was frequented by students from all quarters of the British Isles and the colonies, these measures came to rule medical practice for many years throughout the world. It is certainly true that Colles was influenced by that teaching and he departed little from its principles during his subsequent career in Dublin. Gregory's most abiding monument in the temple of fame is a powder containing rhubarb, magnesia and ginger, which has been perhaps more universally employed than any other pharmacopial preparation.

During the years 1795 to 1797 Colles attended the lecture courses of Andrew Duncan (institutions of medicine), J. Black and T. C. Hope (chemistry and pharmacy), D. Rutherford (botany), A. Monro (anatomy and surgery), Frances Home (materia medica), Alexander Hamilton (midwifery), and J. Allcry (animal economy). During the whole period he was attending clinical lectures and the practice of the Royal Infirmary, and also a three months course at the Edinburgh General Lying-In Hospital. His class tickets for these courses are still preserved. Colles was then no ordinary medical student. He was the product of a famous public school, an arts graduate of an ancient university, and a licentiate of a new but vigorous school of surgery. He had received the best general and medical education that his country could then provide. For him this was now post-graduate training and he absorbed all that was good in the Edinburgh medical scene, and, being by nature tolerant, saw good in all men. He was a prolific reader, both in the university library and in his student digs in Nicholson Street, where his landlady deliberately interrupted his studies, "in case he reads himself into a coffin".

In March 1796 Colles took his seat in the Speculative Society of Edinburgh by virtue of his membership of the College Historical Society of Trinity—incidentally a reciprocity still enjoyed by these famous societies. He regularly attended the weekly meetings and took part in practically all the debates of that vigorous cultural society, until May 1797. In February 1797 he read a paper to the society entitled *The Foundations of Morals*. His stringent financial resources made life frugal in the extreme; sharing digs with a fellow student he was always seeking cheaper accommodation. He cooked his own meals and was ever conscious of the price of foodstuffs, "but as it is necessary to eat, we must buy as well as we can without grumbling". One letter records his pleasure that the "threepenny loaf is larger by one ounce this week". He did not relish the ready salted beef, then the common diet of the poor. "Fish is the standing dish now, for ten pence I got as much good cod which served Whistler (his room-mate) and me three days for our dinner, and it is not impossible but that our landlady also enjoyed some of this frugal though delicious repast. You must know that I have got very fond of fish, so much that nothing prevents my becoming a complete Laplander in diet but a fear of eating too much." "The General Assembly of the Kirk of Scotland is now sitting here, but is not a simple plague but a plague accompanied by a famine. I assure you that the price of mutton was raised two pence a pound on the approach of such a formidable host." He makes many references to the delightful countryside around Edinburgh, which he explored each weekend with his friend, ending up with a meal at an ale house. "We dined on mutton chops, the best I ever tasted, good peas and some fried bacon and bread and butter, but we paid well for all these luxuries, one shilling each—that is twice as dear as our dinner on the Sunday before, for which we only paid six pence each." "For having this day laid aside my winter togs and put on the summer dress my capital landlady could not be restrained, even by the dictates of female modesty, from telling me that I was a very *spry buck*, and recommended to me very strongly to wear hair powder. I need scarcely tell you that, strong as my pride is, it could not prevail on me to go to the expense of six guineas a year, although I was tempted by the assurance of captivating a Scotch Lassy." "As you know that a short cut to fortune was always a wish of mine, you will not be astonished when I tell you of my having joined with Whistler, and purchased the sixteenth of a ticket in this last lottery: but perhaps you will wish to know, did we succeed. We did, but how!

Why, by our ticket having stayed in the wheel for thirty-three days, and then turning up a prize of six pence to each of us. However, we each gained six pence by the lottery and a great many walks to the lottery office to enquire about our ticket." "Tho' I think, with you, that I live very reasonably here, yet I fear very little will be saved for my return, as I propose not to spare any expense which I consider necessary for completing myself in this profession. I would rather live on the Irish dish of *potatoes* and *points*, with a thorough knowledge of my business, than to eat *beef* every day and not know as much as I should of it." On a visit to Edinburgh Castle, where a new barracks was being built, he saw sixteen or seventeen unfortunate French prisoners confined there, who were amusing themselves in playing with and nursing their gaolers' children. He also gives an interesting account of a visit to Holyrood House.

In June 1796, Abraham was host in Edinburgh to his brother, William, who had walked with a friend from London in twelve days, including two days at York. "The young travellers have arrived here. They are both in rude health and the most perfect models of *crops* that Edinburgh can boast of, particularly Kitt. His head I know not to what I can compare, unless to the head of a young bird breaking thro' the shell, the hair lies so smooth and so thin that no one hair does lie above another. I think he will be the leading *crop*, at all events he is the most *knowing* one in this city." William describes this walk in an amusing letter to his mother—"We were sometimes taken for sailors avoiding the press; sometimes for tradesmen out of employment; sometimes for servants out of a place, and sometimes for highwaymen flying from justice. Twice, and twice only, were we mistaken for gentlemen!" In September of that year the two brothers, with two friends, set out to walk to Glasgow, and on the way visited Mr. Dale's cotton mills at Lanark, then employing some eighteen hundred people, including three or four hundred little boys and girls under the age of ten. "At the inn we got a good supper of cold lamb and eggs for eight pence and we paid two pence each for our bed, and indeed the sheets had not been lain in only by a gent from the country! As we were neither proud nor saucy it served us very well until morning, when we thought it smelt rather rank!

William and Cuthbert had got into a dirty flagged room, where they got everything in a most uncomfortable manner at a higher price than our comfortable accommodation, but they had the addition of a whole nation of bugs and surely it is but reasonable that men should pay for their attendants!"

In June 1797 Colles graduated M.D. Edinburgh, after defending a thesis *De Venaesectione* which he dedicated to his brother William and his uncle Richard, and which is still preserved in the Edinburgh University library. Of the 46 graduates of that year there were 14 Irish, 12 English, 7 Scots, 1 "British", 4 Genevans, 2 French, 2 Jamaicans, and 1 each from Barbados, Virgin Islands, Antigua, and Orkney (Islands). The doctorate, as an initial degree, was then an added attraction of Edinburgh, in contrast to the initial bachelor degree of Oxford, Cambridge, and Dublin universities. The examination in Edinburgh, as elsewhere, was conducted entirely in Latin and, not surprisingly, each candidate went to a "grinder" for polishing in that language and in the general conduct of the examination. The custom was for the medical faculty to meet for the examination successively at one another's houses, and for the host to bear the chief brunt of the duty of examining the candidate, which usually lasted some hours. The subsequent acts of the examination consisted of a written commentary on a case drawn up by a professor, and the defence of a thesis. But as these exercises were all written at home and in Latin, they were often the composition of the candidate's "grinder". My colleague, Professor Adams, who translated the Colles M.D. thesis for me, assures me that it was not "grinder's" Latin, and was of a much higher standard, most probably the product of Colles' own classical education.

It is of interest to record that one Irishman graduated M.D. Edinburgh in 1726 and the numbers gradually increased to fifteen in 1800. Of the 800 M.D. degrees awarded there in the last quarter of the eighteenth century, there were 237 Irishmen, 217 Englishmen, 179 Scots and 167 colonials and foreigners. Colles had early decided that this was an unnecessary drain on the manpower, the finances, and the prestige of his country, and that it only required better medical training facilities in Dublin, to reverse the necessity of Irishmen travelling abroad for medical training and degrees. He never departed from this view and the result of his own efforts in developing a medical school at home for his countrymen, received this graceful tribute from "Auld Reekie" forty years later—

> "The Royal College of Surgeons in Ireland is perhaps the most enlightened surgical incorporation in Europe and requires from its members a greater range of accurate knowledge than any other body, excepting the medical faculty of the University of Edinburgh.
>
> *Edinburgh Medical Journal*, 1837."

About June 1797 Colles left Edinburgh for London. It is frequently stated that he walked the entire distance and that he left an account of the journey. The writer is satisfied that no such pedestrian journey took place and agrees with Kirkpatrick that his brother William's reverse journey from London to Edinburgh, of which records exist, has been erroneously accredited to the better known Abraham. Colles had an introduction to Astley Cooper, no doubt from Monro, with whom Cooper worked as a student in Edinburgh for seven months in 1787. Cooper stated that at that time the standard of surgery in London was superior to that taught in Edinburgh, but he learned in Edinburgh an orderly and systematic method of examining and considering the diagnosis and treatment of cases, which he retained throughout life. Cooper's estimate of Monro was—"He grunted like a pig, he was a tolerable lecturer, possessed of a full knowledge of his subject, had much sagacity in practice, was laudably zealous, but was much given to self and to the abuse of others." Cooper, five years older than Colles, was originally apprenticed to his uncle, William Cooper of Guy's Hospital, but later transferred to Cline at St. Thomas's Hospital—both hospitals were then combined in one medical school. Cooper had also attended John Hunter's lectures for several years. Of him he writes—"He was a bad lecturer, his presentation was irksome and devoid of method, and his language obscure. Hunter learned from no man, but from his own observations." Cooper at that time was married to a wealthy wife, was little interested in surgical practice and was

engaged in his monumental work on hernia, which he published
in two volumes in 1804 and 1807, and dedicated to Cline and
Monro respectively. There seems little doubt that Colles helped
in the dissections necessary for that work, although his name
does not appear in its pages, and one is forced to recall G. T.
Bettany's biographical note on Cooper in the *Dictionary of
National Biography*. "He cannot be classed among men of
genius or even of true scientific attainments. His works are not
classic, but they are more than respectable. They are defective
especially from their almost entire omission to refer to the work
of others." Cooper became the leading surgeon in London after
his appointment to Guy's Hospital in 1800, ending with enormous wealth, prestige, a baronetcy, and a statue in St. Paul's
Cathedral among England's heroes. No greater example in
contrasts can be cited than the family lives and careers of
Cooper and Colles, who were for some forty years to lead the
surgical professions in London and Dublin respectively, but, as
is often the case in contrasts, there was an extraordinary degree
of respect and affection between them. They corresponded
frequently, but it is doubtful whether they ever met again.
Colles dedicated his book on the venereal—perhaps his greatest
work, to his friend, Astley Cooper. There is little other information of Colles' sojourn in London, but no doubt during the six
months he "walked the hospitals" there. As he was now away
from Ireland for over two years, and had seen "this sceptre'd
isle" and met "this happy breed of men", he set out for home.

> Such is the patriot's boast where'er we roam
> His first, best country, ever is at home.
>
> Oliver Goldsmith.

Colles returned to Dublin in November, 1797 to find his
country in chaos and on the eve of rebellion. The great eighteenth century, the Age of Reason, ended in the destruction of
the social order in Ireland, England and France. Ireland had
been at peace for a hundred years after William's victory
on the Boyne in 1690 had established the Protestant Ascendancy, but for native Ireland, subjected to a penal code described
by Dr. Johnson as "exceeding in malignance the persecutions

of antiquity", it was a peace of despair. Writing of that century later, the English historian, John Richard Green, states—"It was a period that no Englishman can recall without shame." It is true that the Ascendancy contributed much in culture to Ireland and to the world, and that the vast majority of them were tolerant of and helpful to their Catholic fellow country-men; especially after the failure of the Jacobite Rebellion, when the Irish penal laws were gradually relaxed in practice if not in law. "The important posts of the country, however, were being filled by Englishmen and there was a run of beef-eating, bored, and bigoted nonentities who succeeded each other in dismal and stodgy pomp at Dublin Castle" (Craig). Every Chancellor of Ireland was an Englishman till 1785. Grattan's Parliament in 1782 was initially successful and achieved virtual independence, but it later became unrepresentative and corrupt. Some measures of relief were given to the Roman Catholics in 1793, and more were about to be given by Fitz-william, the new Viceroy in 1795, when he was suddenly recalled. His departure from Dublin was observed as a day of mourning. All hopes of Catholic emancipation now faded. Societies of United Irishmen spread throughout Ireland under a brave leader, Wolfe Tone, deriving their inspiration as well as their republican doctrine from Danton. England was now in a desperate situation with her war with France, and the real rulers of Ireland were the Viceroy and a group of three remarkable men, Clare, Beresford, and Castlereagh. The French landings at Kinsale were unsuccessful on account of weather, and the Franco-Dutch fleet was destroyed at sea by Admiral Duncan. More French aid was promised and a rebellion planned for the following year. This was the Ireland that Colles returned to. He was in desperate straits financially and no doubt had to seek his uncle's help to survive. He took some rooms in Chatham Street and did some general practice, but with the sick poor this was not lucrative. He took over a stable attached to a house in neighbouring King Street and taught some students anatomy and surgery. He gave his services free to the Dispensary for the Sick Poor in Meath Street, in the heart of the "Liberties"—the slum area of the city. But of his first year, November 1797—November 1798, which brought him in a total of £8 16s. 7½d., he writes—"Apparently a trifling sum, yet considering the length of time I was sick and in the country and that it was my first year after my return from Scotland, I do not look on it as dispiriting circumstances that my fees have been so few and so small." The few entries in his fee book reveal both his humour and his courage—"For giving ineffectual advice for deafness— £1 2s. 9d." "For attempting to draw the stump of a tooth." Another, "I know not for what services, unless he may have thought the last fee too small." The month of April, 1799 is marked with the emphatic word "feeless". "For telling him that he was *not* dyspeptic—a guinea." On the other side of the page is the word "hypochondriac". In spite of his courage, there were times which tempted him to take the easy way out and join the armies of Pitt, but Colles loved his country and desired to serve only it. He knew of the injustice meted out to millions of his fellow countrymen and saw the tragedy of the Rebellion, the savagery of the soldiers that suppressed it, the massacre of innocent Protestants, the sectarian character of the revolt, the rise of the Orange Order, and the rebel dead suspended from Carlisle Bridge. It is estimated that in that Rebellion some fifteen thousand lost their lives, sixteen hundred soldiers and eleven thousand rebels were killed in the field, four hundred loyalists were massacred, and two thousand rebels were exiled or hanged. John Kells Ingram, a Fellow of Trinity, was later to make that Rebellion immortal in his *Memory of the Dead*

> "Who fears to speak of ninety-eight?
> Who blushes at the name?
> When cowards mock the patriot's face
> Who hangs his head for shame?
> He's all a knave or half a slave
> Who slights his country thus:
> But a true man, like you, man,
> Will fill your glass with us . . ."

1798 was a tragic year for Colles and his country. His old teacher, William Dease, first professor of surgery in the Surgeons' School and "Father of Irish Surgery", was told that as a

United Irishman he was about to be arrested and tried for treason. Dease died suddenly and probably by his own hand. His colleague, William Lawless, professor of anatomy, was more active in the United Irishmen movement and went "on the run". Escaping to France, he became a brigadier-general in the French forces. With Wolfe Tone, he had an interview with Napoleon, seeking aid for his country, and was not impressed with "Boney", who was surprised that a civilised country like Ireland should still be infested with wolves! Lawless had his foot shot off in an engagement with the British and had his foot amputated by Larrey, the great French surgeon and friend of Napoleon. After the operation Lawless mounted his horse and rode off—he knew what hospital gangrene was. We take leave of him, swimming a river to safety, under a hail of British bullets. His cousin, Lord Cloncurry, himself a prisoner in the Tower for two years, relates with pride his kinsman's exploits, and tells us that were it not for the amputation Lawless would have reached full general's rank in the Army of France. Thomas Wright, superintendent of dissections at the Surgeons' School under Lawless, was likewise active in the rebel movement. He was caught and imprisoned, but having served under Cornwallis at Yorktown, his old chief, now Viceroy of Ireland, had him promptly released. Wright subsequently emigrated to America.

John Fitzgibbon ("Black Jack"), now Lord Clare (and later Earl), Lord Chancellor of Ireland, was the black villain of that period. Clare narrowly escaped assassination at the time of Fitzwilliam's recall. On another occasion Richard Power, Third Baron of the Exchequer, is alleged to have attempted to take the life of Lord Clare with a loaded pistol. Unfortunately failing in this laudable endeavour he set out to Irishtown to commit suicide by drowning which he did. It was remarked by witnesses afterwards that, as the day was wet, he took an umbrella! Clare had the Rebellion put down by force and was constantly seeking out the cells of United Irishmen, then numerous in the city. He arrived at Trinity on a famous Visitation to question all staff and students on their political activities. Whitley Stokes—the father of the great William Stokes, a distinguished fellow of the College, suffered his lordship's displeasure and was demoted. Dozens of students were rusticated on that occasion.

Young Colles in that year, and indeed for many years before, was a constant visitor at the home of his uncle, Richard Colles, a barrister at 135 St. Stephen's Green, and depended on him for financial support; but all these debts were later repaid in full. Richard had risen to considerable eminence in his profession, but his career suffered through the enmity of Lord Clare, who unrelentingly revenged himself for some stricture on his conduct which Richard had published. He is said to have been a remarkably small man, and as sometimes happens in similar circumstances, contracted a close friendship with a singularly tall barrister named Mahaffy, and being inseparable companions and constantly seen together in public, they became the object to their brother barristers of many witticisms and at least one poetical effusion. There was a story told of what occurred on one occasion when they appeared in court on opposite sides of the same case. Mr. Mahaffy addressed the court first, and when he concluded his remarks the judge said, "Please sit down, Mr. Mahaffy". He replied, "I am sitting down, my lord". Colles then began to speak. "When you address the court, Mr. Colles" said the judge, "you should stand up". "I am standing on the seat, my lord" he replied. For a time Richard Colles was a widower, his wife dying in 1793. Of their five children, four died in infancy. He remarried, however, in 1796, and was a father of six more children, of whom four died in infancy. He was ever a generous and good-natured man, who resigned a judgeship on the day of his appointment, at the request of his brother-in-law, Denis George, next in nomination to the vacant bench. He was particularly generous to Abraham and his brothers, and his house in Dublin was always open to them. Richard's son, Edward, like his father, was a barrister and equally distinguished. He became Chief Justice of Sierra Leone and on returning home some years later he became librarian of the Royal Dublin Society, in which post, according to family records, he was especially noted for his kindness to student readers. According to the R.D.S. records, however, his career there caused the Society very anxious moments, as on one occasion when a distinguished reader was addressed as "a half-blooded mongrel".

In his uncle's home Abraham would have learned of the career of Christopher Colles, his father's cousin, then in the United States. Christopher, like his uncle William of Abbeyvale, was a man of varied talent, untiring energy, and considerable genius. As an engineer and architect he was for a short while Director of Inland Navigation of the Shannon before he emigrated with his cousin John to America in 1771. He was the first to propose a waterway linking up the Great Lakes with the Atlantic via the Mohawk River, and in the great celebrations in New York in 1825 to mark the completion of the scheme, the effigy of Colles was borne with dignity in that vast procession. In 1789 his great classic, *A survey of the roads of the United States*, appeared, and this was reprinted in 1961 by the Harvard University Press. His career, however, showed great fluctuations in fortune, and at one time he was so poor that he was marketing mouse traps. He believed in signs as firmly as Napoleon and was fixed in the opinion that he was born under an unlucky star. "Had he been brought up to the trade of a hatter", he was wont to say, "mankind would have come into the world without heads". Always cheerful and good humoured, he met fate with dignity. He was given a state funeral, and his memory is honoured as one of the worthiest pioneers of American progress. His name appears in the *American Dictionary of Biography*.

In June 1799, Philip Woodroffe died, and on July 26th of the same year Abraham Colles, now aged twenty-six, was appointed to succeed his old master as resident surgeon at Dr. Steevens' Hospital. This, for Colles, was the turning point in his career, and for the hospital the most important appointment ever made in its long history. Colles was given a salary of £55 per annum for his administrative duties and £5 per annum in lieu of furniture. He had free accommodation in the hospital and no restriction on private practice, either within or without the hospital. He had an equal share of the beds with the assistant surgeons, Boyton and Obré. The post was certainly not strictly resident, as Colles had an address at 10 Pitt Street and later at 71 Dame Street during that period. On 4th

November 1799 Colles was elected a member* of the Royal
College of Surgeons in Ireland, which rank now entitled him
to take apprentices. His earnings for that year, ending 1799,
were £178 4s. 4½d. "This is a very great sum of money for my
second year's practice; compare it with the previous' year's
total and the comparison is very flattering."

As the fortunes of Colles rose, those of his country sank
lower. Pitt and his Parliament realised that the Irish Parliament could no longer govern a country torn in hatred and
discord after the Rebellion, and that the Union of Parliaments
was an Imperial necessity. Few in Ireland desired such a
Union, apart from that small ruling clique who saw in it the
means of destroying any further Catholic hopes of emancipation.
Lord Clare, who had the ear of the King, reminded him of his
coronation oath, which became a fixation in the mind of that
dull old monarch. Pitt, who was unable to keep his promises
to the Roman Catholics at the time of the Union, instead of
resigning, might well have reminded the King that Parliament
which had in 1689 imposed this oath on the King could also
in 1800 relieve him from it. "How the Union was effected by
offices, pensions, threats of dismissal, peerages, and the buying
out of the rest makes one of the most unpleasing pictures of
history and disgusted even Cornwallis and those who did the
buying" (Curtis). As for Clare, now an Earl, he suited everyone's convenience by dying in bed two years later, and received
a nation's tribute in showers of curses and dead cats on his
coffin. Counsellor Jeremiah Keller, when approached by a
deputation of the bar to know whether he would attend Lord
Clare's funeral replied, "I shall certainly attend his funeral
with the greatest pleasure imaginable". Lady Clare was made
of better stuff. She could scarcely be otherwise, as the sister of
playboy Buck Whaley. A certain Doctor Richard Twiss after
paying a brief visit to Ireland wrote his impressions of his tour
and in these he cast some illiberal reflexions on Irish womenfolk. A Dublin manufacturer of earthenware had the doctor's
countenance painted on the bottom of chamberpots—"with
his mouth and eyes open ready to receive the libation". For

*The term "fellow" was substituted for "member" in the 1844 Charter.

these wares Lady Clare, in the aristocratic humour of the time, composed the following motto—

> Here you may behold a liar,
> Well deserving of hell-fire.
> Everone who likes may p . . .
> Upon the learned Doctor T . . .

And now with Dublin referring to these vessels as a "Twiss", it is a convenient time to take leave of the eighteenth century, the Age of Reason, and the Age of Scandal that followed it.

CHAPTER 4

Professor and Surgeon

"Be assured, that no man can know his profession
perfectly, who knows nothing else; and that he
who aspires to eminence in any particular science
must first acquire the habit of philosophizing on
matters of science in general."*

Abraham Colles: *A Treatise on Surgical Anatomy*, 1811.

A few months after his election to membership of the Royal
College of Surgeons in Ireland in 1799, Colles was elected an
assistant in January 1800, elected a censor, i.e. examiner, in
1801, and in 1802 at the early age of 29 he was elected president
of the College. In July 1802 James Cleghorn resigned the chair
of anatomy and chirurgery at Trinity. The younger Cleghorn,
who had succeeded to his uncle's chair in 1790, being "appointed at 10 o'clock at night,"was, like his Edinburgh counterpart, Alexander Monro *Tertius*, an academic failure. A
physician, with little interest in anatomy and surgery, and even
less ability to teach it, he did little to develop the Trinity school.
For some time Cleghorn's duties as professor were being discharged by Professor William Hartigan, who was professor of
anatomy and surgery in the Surgeons' School (1789–1799), and
had taught Colles as a student in that school. Hartigan, one of
the original members appointed by the surgeons under their new
charter, had no university degree and Trinity awarded him an
honorary M.D. when he was a locum professor there. In 1802
Colles applied for the Trinity chair, with Hartigan, his old
teacher, as opponent. Colles was defeated, and in the following
year took action in law against Trinity in an endeavour to
have the election declared void on the grounds that Hartigan,
having only an honorary degree in medicine, was not qualified

*Quoted by Maurice B. Strauss—Familiar Medical Quotations. 1968.

to deliver clinical lectures. The court, however, decided against him and never again did Colles seek for any post in Trinity. Trinity at that time was not yet ready for change and even under the second School of Physic Act of 1800 they were still loath to advance their school. Hartigan, a kind old gentleman, suited their requirements. Fond of cats, which he took in his overcoat pockets when visiting his patients, he amused himself and his Trinity students till his death in 1812. His widow writing to his successor, Macartney, in answer to an enquiry with regard to the financial prospects of this chair, said that "the income had lately fallen greatly because so many of the College lads from whom the salary is levied generally went into the Army or took to surgery before the second year expired, and it is from the pupils of that long-standing that the professor is paid. The exertions of the College of Surgeons to draw all the pupils they could to their school, as also the number of junior lecturers, reduce our income very much, and these last three years they did not produce altogether above £100 per annum. If I were to advise you as a friend it would be never to wear out your lungs for such a paltry sum. I am convinced it shortened my dear H's life and it was not my fault that he did not resign it years back." Mrs. Hartigan was not, however, entirely disinterested, as she and Wilmot, who was expected to succeed her husband, had come to an arrangement whereby Wilmot's salary would be transferred to her. Trinity did rise again and it was the appointment in 1813 of this man, James Macartney, that shook them out of their complacency and "made" their School.

Meanwhile, Colles having failed to obtain the Trinity chair in 1802, had not long to wait, as in September 1804 on the resignation of Professor John Halahan, he was appointed to the chair of anatomy and physiology and to the chair of surgery in the Surgeons' School. In both chairs he had as co-professor, Richard Dease, who succeeded his distinguished father in 1798. In 1804 a hundred students attended the anatomy classes of the Surgeons' School; these numbers increased rapidly and averaged 250 during the Colles regime. Colles now went back to that little building styled the Surgeons' Theatre in Mercer Street, at the back of the hospital founded by Mary Mercer in 1734, to begin his career as professor. The building had little changed since his student days, although it had acquired an adjacent outhouse, giving it direct access to Glover's Alley, so that bodies could be admitted more secretly into the College premises. The debts on the building had now been paid by government grants. Larger premises were an immediate necessity on account of overcrowding, and in this the government was again sympathetic; it being realised that the vast majority of the students of the School were only seeking that diploma qualifying them for the armies of Pitt. Colles was appointed to a committee of the College in the following year to advise on a new building, and a new site was procured for £4,000 at the corner of York Street/St. Stephen's Green. This was part of a Quaker burial ground not then in use, and on this a new home for the College was built between 1806 and 1810. This was a two storeyed granite building, surmounted by a triangular pediment, and containing accommodation for the president and his council, a large dissecting room, theatre, museum, and library for the College school. The government contributed no less than £29,000 and the College emerged wealthy, commodious and comfortable—the council room carpet alone costing £48 5s. 3d.

"Erinensis" (subsequently identified as an Irishman, named Dr. Herris Greene), in a series of brilliant, satirical, but mostly scurrilous letters to *The Lancet* (1823–1830) on the Dublin medical scene, wrote of this new College.

"A neat little structure which suddenly arose from the site of the Quakers' burial ground at the corner of York Street/St. Stephen's Green. On the 17th March, 1806 the usual ceremony of laying the foundation stone was performed by the Lord Lieutenant, and as it now stands it reminds one very strongly of the appearance of these people whose relics it has sacriligiously supplanted—it looks for all the world like the genius of Quakerism personified in stone. Solid and substantial, no gew-gaw of the sculptor's art disfigures the simplicity of its style. With a facade of Portland stone resting on a basement of mountain granite and supporting a cornice terminating in an angle on top, it stands, the pride of Irish

surgery and the terror of many a candidate whose fate
depends on its decrees."

But even this new building could not accommodate the numbers of students attending Colles' classes, and fifteen years later
(1825) the present magnificent building, incorporating the old,
was built on an extended site and completed in 1827. No longer
could "Erinensis" state that "no gew-gaw of the sculptor's art
disfigures the simplicity of its style", as the pediment of the new
building supports three majestic figures, each seven feet in
height, representing the Greek deities Asclepius, Athena and
Hygieia, while the tympanum is charged with the Royal Arms
sculptured in relief. This College is in fact the monument to
Colles; it was his success as a teacher by attracting so many
students that made its extension a necessity, and it is the same
College, apart from some internal structural alterations, that
we know today.

Let "Erinensis" in his amusing satire describe the scene of
that lecture theatre.

"But the bell rings—Mr. Colles' carriage is at the gate—
the benches fill—confusion in all its fantastic forms of juvenile
levity prevails throughout the scene. The whole artillery of
confectionery, from canister lozenges to the heavy grape shot
of spice nuts, is flying on all sides, while other aspirants for
anarchial reputation eagerly contend for the aromatic
ammunition. On another side, some musical amateur
amuses the audience with the fashionable song or quadrille
of the day. Thus everyone contributes something to increase
this scene of unphilosophical tumult. Here I must cease—
the folding doors open and in hurries Mr. Colles with a slip
of paper twisted round his index finger—a simultaneous
burst of applause greets his welcome entry, but modestly
declining the honour intended him, he instantly proceeds
without even returning the salute, Gentlemen, at our last
meeting," etc. etc. Some 250 students settle themselves to
listen. "Their mere appearance", continues "Erinensis", "is
our present concern, and as they sit in the living panorama
before us, they do not much accord with notions which might
be formed of a body of medical students. The same number

of young men taken from the various counting houses or haberdashers' shops, through town, would present as much of the elements of genius, as much of the deep traces of thought, as much of everything else which gives a studious character to the countenance, as this blue-frocked, black-booted, black-socked, Wellington-booted assemblage of medical dandies. Gold rings, broad and bright, glitter here and there among the artful labours of the friseur, as the hand supports the head, thrown into an attitude of mental abstraction; steel guard chains, often without watches to protect, sparkle almost on every breast, and quizzing glasses hang gracefully pendant from each neck; in short, the whole paraphernalia of puppyism are displayed here in the greatest possible profusion." The lecturer describes in rapid succession symptoms and treatment of several cases, illustrating the day's theme. "In this dogmatic effusion, books, authors, and authorities are all run over, to arrive at the one arbitrary and everlasting conclusion, the truth is, gentlemen, these men know nothing of the matter. . . . He is never at a loss for appropriate terms to express his meaning, though he evidently labours to comprise a great deal in a short space, the very effort is often at the expense of offensive diffuseness. Having promised some general principles, fiction or reality supplies him with a case. This offspring of his fancy he places in as many different points of view as his invention can suggest. He seems to think that his observations should all be original, and they usually are so, merely because he wishes they should differ from any other authority. Contrast is another weapon which Mr. Colles wields with peculiar dexterity. For this purpose he disinters from the grave of antiquated practice some absurd proposals, and placing these beside some improvement or discovery in modern surgery, it is quite amusing to hear him comment upon the ludicrous comparison, and to see with what gusto he enjoys the imaginary triumph. It is only on these occasions that his leucophlegmatic countenance ever betrays any symptoms of internal agitation, or that a rush of the vital current of the heart diffuses a blush over the habitual marble-like paleness of his face. Having seized, however, on some unfortunate theorist, a momentary flash of indignation lights up his rigid features and, like one of these birds peculiar to the Irish shores, that soars into the clouds to destroy its prey by letting it fall on the rocks below, he gradually poises himself upon the wings of self-sufficiency and fancied superiority, until his vengeance, from exertion, becomes expended, and then dashes out his victim's brains upon some rugged commonplace of contumulous reprobation."

Colles' lectures were not only fluent, but they were enlivened by practical anecdotes, *bon mots* and *double entendres*, with which he sent his hearers into roars of laughter. "Erinensis" was not one who lightly bestowed praise, yet he states that Colles was then the greatest figure in the College, and in a series of some thirty profiles of the Dublin School he gives Colles No. 1 place, and continues:

"Without many books, and paying less attention to their contents, he is still the laborious, shrewd, observing, matter-of-fact, and practical surgeon. As an operator, he has many equals and some superiors, but in advice, from long experience, and a peculiar tact of discovering the hidden causes of disease, he has scarcely a rival."

Anatomy has ever been regarded as the very basis of the surgeon's art and Colles naturally directed his full energies to the subject on assuming the College chairs. He had to alter the teaching of the subject in Dublin, which at that time was almost Vesalian in method. He was concerned with the provision of an adequate supply of anatomical material for growing numbers of students at a time which unfortunately coincided with the "resurrectionist" activities and the grave public disquiet which followed their gruesome trade. Finally, he and his College laid a successful protest against an Act of Parliament which required the bodies of executed murderers to be handed over to the surgeons for dissection, which for Ireland, with its high incidence of political murders, had dangerous implications. For proper appreciation of this the reader may wish to be reminded of the evolution of anatomy.

Human anatomy, as a subject for scientific study, began in

the great Alexandrian school of medicine (330–280 B.C.) under its celebrated teachers Herophilus and Erasistratus—the "founders of human anatomy". Human dissection was expressly forbidden by the Greeks, and in latter-day Rome, where practically all its medical practitioners were Greeks, the same limitations prevailed. It is a curious reflexion on the absence of humanity among the Roman Quirites that they consistently regarded the practice of medicine as being beneath them, and the "greedy little Greeks", as Juvenal called them, collected large fees in the mercenary and unsavoury practice of the day. Galen's uncomplimentary opinion of his professional brethren is expressed in his caustic aphorism, "between robbers and physicians lies this difference only, that the former's misdeeds are in the mountains, but the latter's in Rome itself".

Galen, a Greek, born in 130 A.D. at Pergamum, was the most important medical authority in antiquity after Hippocrates. He studied anatomy and surgery at Smyra and Alexandria before coming to Rome, where he attracted the esteem of the Emperor, Marcus Aurelius. He was a diligent and accurate anatomist, although his dissections were mainly on animals; chiefly pigs and apes. He discovered and named the cranial nerves and demonstrated the flow of urine from the kidneys to the bladder, and produced aphonia by division of the recurrent laryngeal nerves. He described the clinical signs of tetanus very accurately, and it is from his text we use today such terms as "opisthonus", "ischuria", "oedema", "hydrocele", and many others, all of Greek derivation. Galen's death in Sicily in 200 A.D. was the downfall of anatomy in ancient times, and from that time on its study languished in neglect and obscurity for more than a thousand years, for his knowledge of anatomy was accepted as final up to the time of Vesalius. During that long period also, the rise of Muhammad (570–633 A.D.) brought about a truly dark age in anatomy and surgery in Europe, Alexandria, after nine hundred years of learning, perished in flames in the middle of the seventh century, and for the next hundred years the hordes of Islam spread westward along the African shores to establish a firm footing in Spain. To this Arab influence in Europe we are however under an enormous debt. They gave us our numerals, algebra, trigonometry, and the use of the pendulum: they taught us the identification of alcohol, potash, silver nitrate, corrosive sublimate and sulphuric acid. They introduced paper, which secret they had learned from the Chinese. As in Greece of old, the rules of Islam forbade human dissection: the Koran denouncing as unclean that person who defiles a corpse. Hence, Arabic anatomy was largely acquired by translations from the text of Galen, and the Alexandrian anatomists. Arab society protected itself from surgical enthusiasm by the rule that before operating on the Faithful the tyro must first have operated successfully on three unbelievers! Surgeons should remember that it was this Arab aversion to the shedding of blood of the Faithful that led to the introduction of the cautery. With the Greek predominance, and in the Roman Empire, there was no distinction between the physician and the surgeon. Arabic physicians were the first to inculcate the doctrine of the inferiority of the surgical branch of the healing art, which persisted for centuries after the expulsion of the Moslems from Western Europe, and the practice of surgery was relegated to the barbers and strolling mountebanks. From the Hippocratic conception of surgery as the true right arm of medicine, its devotees steadily sank to the most menial position, and Arab influence was primarily responsible for the lack of surgical development between the seventh and twelfth centuries.

Human anatomy was re-born in the Italian schools. In Bologna, the oldest University in Europe, there was a medical faculty in 1260 and Mondino, the first of the Italian anatomists, published his text-book there in 1315; a little volume which served as "the small Cunningham", or more correctly "the small Galen" for several centuries. Practically all the pre-renaissance anatomists were successors of Mondino in the chair at Bologna and woodcuts of the period show the professors literally in their chairs, perched high and reading from their texts, while below them in the amphitheatres some menial barber-surgeon was demonstrating the parts on human and animal material. It is doubtful whether the great men ever descended from their chairs to dissect for themselves. The artists were next to develop anatomy, and there is evidence that Verrochio, Mantegna, Leonardo, Cellini, and Michaelangelo all practised human dissection, wielding the scalpel that they might the better wield brush and chisel, before ever Vesalius set foot in Italy. As artists, concerned with the natural reproduction of the body in action, the chief object of their study was the surface musculature, neglected by the professional anatomist— with the delineation of the hand, the contour of the shoulder, and above all, stimulated by improved access to Greek sources, with the determination of the true canon of proportions. Had not da Vinci's famous drawings handed to his faithful Francesco Melzi been lost for about three centuries, the title of father of our modern anatomy might well have gone to the Florentine and not to Vesalius.

Andreas Witting or Wesele whose name had been latinised to Vesalius, was born near Brussels in 1515, and was later to take the road south to Italy and inaugurate there the golden age of anatomy in the great re-awakening of learning known as the renaissance. Graduating from Louvain in philosophy, he migrated to Paris where du Bois—known to us as Jacobus Sylvius (1478–1555) was reading the text of Galen to large numbers of students and teaching anatomy from "fragments of dogs' limbs". Sylvius omitted the difficult parts of anatomy from his lectures, and if he found any anatomical structure which did not conform to Galen's description, he alleged that the human body must have changed since Galen's time! Sylvius of Paris was not liberal in his judgment of the work of others. He strongly disapproved of the anatomical discoveries of his pupil Vesalius and even spoke of him, not as Vesalius, but as Vesanus (madman), whose "pestilential breath poisons Europe". Incidentally it was not this Sylvius of Paris, but a namesake Franciscus Sylvius (1614–1672) of Leiden who described the cerebral fissure in 1641 and the cerebral aqueduct c. 1650. Dissatisfied with opportunity for human dissection in Paris, Vesalius left for Padua, the "child of Venice", and was appointed professor. After five years of strenuous work in the dissecting room the famous *De humani corporis fabrica* was produced for the world in 1543. Vesalian anatomy was based wholly on human dissection and the masterpiece illustrated most probably by his fellow countryman, Joannes Stephanus of Calcar, a pupil of Titian, was one of the relevations of the renaissance. Thus, Vesalius became the new founder of anatomy, and to him and to his successors, Fallopius and Fabricus at Padua, men flocked to see the new anatomy. John Caius brought it back to the Barbers' Company in London and to Cambridge, and Peter Pavius took it over the hills to Leiden. It was to Padua that William Harvey went some seventy years later to study the new anatomy for five years under Fabricus. Later his famous manuscript bore the date 1616, although *De Motu Cordis* was not published until 1628 at Frankfurt. In this Harvey bridged an enormous gap in knowledge. The teaching of Galen on the blood circulation was unchallenged by all, including the great Vesalius, for well over a thousand years, but the "septal pores" were now to be swept away for ever in Harvey's immortal discovery of the circulation. Harvey thus takes his place with Galen, Mondino and Vesalius as one of the great four names in the story of anatomy.

Early anatomy was almost entirely confined to the body cavities, with neglect of the limbs. With Vesalius the whole body was dissected and displayed by systems, e.g. in a limb the whole musculature was dissected, in another limb the blood vessels or nerves, and so on. This systematic anatomy was that taught by the Hunters, the Monros, and by Hartigan and Lawless in Dublin. However complete and perfect in display it was not only wasteful of material, but more important, it did not provide the surgeon with the necessary knowledge of the exact relationship of such structures as bone, muscle, nerves and blood vessels to one another. Surgeons required their anatomy to be topographical or applied; this type of anatomy was developed by Pierre Dionis, Jean-Louis Petit, and Marie Bichat in Paris, John Bell in Edinburgh, Astley Cooper in Guy's Hospital, James Macartney, then at St. Bartholomew's Hospital, and now by Abraham Colles in Dublin. Anatomy was now to be subservient to the surgery course which was the reversal of the Edinburgh method where, under Alexander Monro *Secundus*, surgery was dealt with at the tail end of the anatomy course. This surgical anatomy of Colles, and continued by his successors, was the anatomy of the Dublin schools for many decades, and it was really in the closing decades of the nineteenth century that anatomy once again became a subject *per se* under Daniel John Cunningham.

The only legal method of obtaining anatomical material for

dissection was use of the bodies of executed murderers. The Barber Surgeons of Edinburgh in their Seill of Cause in 1505 were allowed one such body per annum for dissection. This also appears to have been the practice at Padua, as we know that Vesalius used to plead with the judge not to sentence the man to quartering, as this would limit his subsequent dissection. In 1541 Henry VIII gave to the Barber Surgeons of London the right to receive annually the bodies of four executed criminals, a privilege later extended to other corporations. The first record of a dissection of a malefactor in Dublin was that performed at at the College of Physicians in 1672 when Thomas Proby and Sir Patrick Dun were present. Under an Act of Parliament, 1752 (George II) styled "For better preventing the horrid crime of murder" the practice became universal. This Act stated—"In order that some terror and peculiar mark of infamy be added to the punishment of death, it was laid down that the bodies of all executed murderers were to be handed over to the appropriate surgeon to be dissected and anatomized." The Royal College of Surgeons in Ireland made use of this act in 1788 in an endeavour to obtain some funds for their College when they refused a body from the sheriff—"the College regret it is not in their power to comply with the act by receiving the body, as the Government has not yet enabled them to procure a hall for public dissection". Heartrending scenes took place in the court as the condemned man pleaded with his judge not to be anatomized. There were certainly some grounds for their fears. In 1650, Ann Green was charged, unjustly it seems, for the murder of her newborn illegitimate child and was hanged at Oxford. In the dissecting room her body showed signs of life and was revived by Petty and Willis (of the arterial circle). The scholars of Oxford made a collection for her, she married, had a family, and lived happily ever after. In 1740 a hanged youth of sixteen, named Duill, also came to life when laid out for dissection in the Barber Surgeons' Hall in London. He was reprieved, transported, and changing his name to Deverell, became a prosperous merchant. Appalling scenes were witnessed at the scaffold as howling mobs of relatives and friends tried to rescue the body from the soldiery on its way to the dissecting rooms. The London College of Surgeons introduced some pageantry into this ghastly enactment of the law. Hiring a house close to Newgate, their president arrayed in full court dress, awaited the bodies on the first floor to the accompaniment of, "the shouts of the crowd below, the rumbling of the cart, and the heavy tramp of the hangman on the stairs. The executioner, coarsely dressed, entered with a body on his back, which he let fall with a heavy thud on the table. The president made a small incision over the sternum and then bowed to the hangman." In Dublin the witticisms of the hangman were much quoted and relished. One, Tom Galvin, would almost cry with disappointment if anyone got a reprieve, exclaiming "It's a hard thing to be taking the bread out of the mouth of an old man like me". On another occasion, when a felon named O'Brien, lingered over his devotions, Galvin said, "Mr. O'Brien, long life to you, make haste wid your prayers, de people is getting tired under the swing-swong." Years later (1830) when Colles was again president of his College, a remarkable and spirited motion was proposed by Crampton against this obnoxious act of parliament. "It is calculated to excite in the minds of the ignorant feelings of hatred and disgust towards the surgical profession because it associates the surgeon with the executioner in the performance of the most odious and degrading of all offices." This protest of the Irish College was partly responsible for the repeal of this act of parliament two years later. The act really was not of much use, for even if the bodies of all executed murderers were conveyed to the anatomical schools, their numbers probably did not exceed an annual average of 38 in England and Wales— no figures for Ireland are available. In practice, therefore, there was but one way of obtaining bodies for dissection, namely by stealing them from graveyards. Vesalius himself admitted doing so and all anatomists since that time received their supplies from that source, although few admitted it. Dease, Hartigan, and Lawless were all skilled in anatomy when the Dublin surgeons received their charter, and must have received their training in small dissecting rooms with supplies from graveyards. At first, strong iron railings around graves, mortsafes, watch towers, watchmen, and vigilant relatives protected the dead, although there were occasional scuffles, free fights, and even murders between the rival parties. Later, as the demand for more subjects grew, the activity was no longer confined to medical students and dissecting-room attendants. It became an actual trade, employing some sixty "resurrectionists" or "sack-em up men" in Dublin alone. They were unhindered in their gruesome activities in lonely graveyards, such as Kilgobbin and Killester, but the main centre of their activity was the huge graveyard known as "*Bully's Acre*"—named after the numerous rowdies and bullies interred there, situated at Kilmainham, and also known as the Hospital Fields. This burial ground was not well guarded, which mattered little, as the watchmen, gravediggers, sextons and undertakers were all in league with "resurrectionists" and the latter not infrequently acted as assistants to undertakers.

> "By day it was his trade to go,
>   Sending his black coach to and fro:
> And sometimes at the Gate of Woe
>   With emblems suitable,
> He stood with brother mutes to show
>   That life is mutable.
> But long before they passed the ferry,
>   The dead, that he had helped to bury,
> He sack's (he had a sack to carry) the bodies
>   off in.
> In fact, he let them have a very short fit of
>   coffin."

It was calculated that some 1500 bodies yearly were robbed from *Bully's Acre* and Dublin's 500 medical students were well provided for. There was bound to be some carelessness in this, as on one occasion when a partially dissected limb was found floating in the Liffey. An inquest having been held, the coroner wrote to the College, who resolved "that the thanks of the College be returned to Alderman Stammer for his polite and able communication and that he be informed that they take the same into their most serious consideration". Colles was advised to take every precaution. There is, however, no record that he or his College did anything to prevent the College premises being used as a warehouse by the "resurrectionists" for their

home and export market. On one occasion a College porter
was murdered and two others nearly so by mobs seeking a stolen
body. Subjects were supplied to the Dublin Schools at a cost
of about thirty shillings, but fetched ten times that price in
London and Edinburgh, which each now had some 900 students. A lucrative export market developed, and "innocent"
cargoes labelled "Salted Herring" and "Irish Cheddar" were
landed on the Ayrshire coast, in Leith, and Liverpool. On one
occasion a poor beggar choked to death on a crust outside St.
Thomas' Hospital in London. The body was taken into the
hospital by a passing stranger, who emerged saying he got a
good price for "his brother's body". James Syme visited Dublin
as a young man in 1826 to arrange supplies of bodies for his
dissecting room. After visiting Dr. Steevens' Hospital he was
amazed at the high standard of surgery practised there by
Colles, Wilmot and Cusack, which determined him to begin
forthwith his surgical career in Edinburgh. "Resurrectionist"
activities were also rampant in Edinburgh and we have already
referred to it at the time of Alexander Monro *Primus* in 1725.
In London, Astley Cooper dealt openly with the "resurrectionists", as the Hunter brothers did before him. Cooper was later
to state publicly, "there is no person, let his station in life be
what it may, whom if I were disposed to dissect I would not
obtain. The law only enhances the price and does not prevent
the exhumation." Macartney of Trinity, who also dealt direct
with the "resurrectionists", attacked the hypocrisy of the
Dublin public in a letter to the press: "I do not think that the
upper and middle classes have understood the effects of their
own conduct when they take part in impeding the progress of
dissection, nor does it seem wise to discountenance the practice
by which many of them are supplied with artificial teeth and
hair. Very many of the upper ranks carry in their mouths teeth
which have been buried in the Hospital Fields." Macartney
in 1828 suggested a better and more noble method of obtaining
bodies for dissection, and in the School of Anatomy in Trinity
there is a document signed by him, and some 277 others, including many distinguished scientists of the period.

"We whose names are hereunto affixed, being convinced that

the study of anatomy is of the utmost value to mankind, inasmuch as it illustrates various branches of natural and moral science, and constitutes the very basis of the healing art; and believing that the erroneous opinions and the vulgar prejudices which prevail with regard to dissections, will be most effectually removed by practical example: do hereby deliberately and solemnly express our desire that, at the usual period after death, our bodies, instead of being interred, should be devoted by our surviving friends to the more rational, benevolent, and honourable purpose of explaining the structure, functions and diseases of the human body."

We will meet Macartney again.

Meanwhile the "resurrectionist" period ended abruptly and in ghastly fashion in Edinburgh. Two debased Irishmen, Burke and Hare, thought of an easier way of obtaining bodies—they murdered by suffocation some sixteen "Daft Jamies" and others of the underworld, disposing of their bodies to the dissection rooms. Burke was hanged in public in January 1829 and Hare, escaping the same penalty by turning King's evidence, heard the shouts of the frenzied mob—"Burke him", and a new verb being added to our language. Warburton, the English Home Secretary, immediately introduced an anatomy bill into the Commons. The Lords, headed by the Archbishop of Canterbury, were sufficiently strong to defeat it; prejudice and ignorance were not confined to the masses. Three years later, three "resurrection" men, Bishop, Williams and May, murdered a 14 years old Italian boy in London and attempted to sell his body to the anatomists of King's College. Bishop and Williams were tried and executed, May was reprieved and transported for life. This shocking murder, almost at the very gates of Westminster, succeeded in awakening the legislators from an apathy out of which the pleas of the teachers, the exposures in the lay press, and the vitriolic pen of Thomas Wakley had failed to stir them. With the passage of Warburton's second anatomy act (1832) the days of the "resurrection" men were over. Their vocation, evil as it had been, was no longer a necessity. The disclosures at the Edinburgh trial of Burke and Hare destroyed the career of Robert Knox, one of Edinburgh's greatest anatomists. He was unlucky in that the body of the last victim was traced to his dissecting room. Hounded, abused and subjected to numerous ballads* he was forced to leave his city and his career. In Dublin, Colles was very fortunate to have escaped similar consequences of the "resurrectionist" activities, and like Burke's paramour Nelly "was out of the scrape". Incidentally, George A. Little was incorrect in stating that one of Colles' sons, a medical student, was shot dead during "resurrectionist" activities; all of Colles' six sons have now been accounted for.

The peace that followed the Napoleonic wars brought with it trade depression and a marked increase in the cost of living. People now began thinking how the existing affairs could be improved. "Reconstruction" became the order of the day. In everything related to the profession of medicine there was ample room for improvement. The regulation and control of practitioners was extremely lax, and in the teaching of those who sought to become practitioners there was a complete want of uniformity among the schools of medicine. Medical graduates of Oxford and Cambridge considered themselves superior to all other medical men, although there was little or no teaching of medicine in their medical schools. In London, the physicians and surgeons were controlled respectively by their Royal Colleges, whose licentiates alone could practise in the city. The great medical school of Edinburgh University suffered considerably from the laxity with which degrees were granted by some of the Scottish universities. Practically anyone could obtain a degree by purchase from Aberdeen and St. Andrews universities, and the value of the Scottish diplomas was lowered accordingly. In Ireland, the School of Physic in Trinity and the Surgeons' School of the Royal College of Surgeons were trying to raise the standard of medical education, but their efforts were hampered by the ease with which students could obtain qualifications in the sister countries. Medical practitioners throughout the three kingdoms, weighed down as they were by adverse economic conditions looked in vain for help to the

---

* "Doun the close and up the stairs,
But and ben wi' Burke and Hare,
Burke's the butcher, Hare's the thief,
Knox the man that buys the beef."

chartered medical corporations, the control of which was largely
in the hands of a few consultants in London, Edinburgh
and Dublin. But these corporations, entrenched safely, as they
believed, behind their charters, resisted strenuously every
effort made to better the lot of the general medical practitioner.
The position of these corporations might have been well-nigh
impregnable, had they been able to keep their houses in order.
There was laxity in the observance of their obligations, a laxity
which in some instances amounted almost to corruption, and
this weakness was well known to those who were leading the
attack against them.   In England, Thomas Wakley founded
The Lancet in 1823, to fight the abuses in the profession, a
fight characterised by incidents of which both parties might
well have been ashamed, and the accounts of it read more like
the description of a drunken row at Billingsgate than of an
argument amongst the members of a learned profession.
Wakley, with all the scurrility of which he was a past master,
attacked all and sundry who opposed him, no matter what their
position, and the leading physicians and surgeons of London did
not consider it beneath their dignity to fight him with his own
weapons. Dublin also had its pioneers in medical reform in
Jacob and Carmichael, but their activities were within the
profession and did not involve the public, as Wakley's un-
ashamedly did. Wakley encroached on the Irish medical scene
by his employment of "Erinensis". In these articles Colles was
often singled out for his failure to project himself as a leader and
to reform his profession. Colles ignored these strictures, as he
was already leading the surgeons of Ireland by education and
example into a profession of dignity and respectability, as
Georges Mareschal had done in Paris a century before. Nor was
Colles upset by the taunt that Dublin did not possess a surgeon
of the daring of a Cooper. This referred to the dramatic ligation
of the abdominal aorta by Astley Cooper in 1817, and his reply
when asked whether he would do it again, "yes, to-morrow, if
I had the opportunity, for I shall never be swayed or ruled by
other people, by those who know nothing about the matter: I
should listen to them as much as I would to the buzzing of a
gnat or the hissing of a goose". This goose, like her famous
ancestors of Juno who by their timely warning saved the

Capitol, may have been warning the great Cooper that surgical daring need not be reckless.

London, in 1826, had a population of some 1,200,000, served by 174 physicians, 1,000 surgeons, and 2,000 apothecaries; and there was a curious comparison with Paris, of 800,000 inhabitants, where the figures were 600, 128 and 131 respectively (Duncan). The London surgeons were separated from the Barber Surgeons Company in 1745, but the new Company of Surgeons were little more than a mere separation of surgeons from barbers. The Company was bound by the bye-laws of the old joint Company and although new bye-laws were approved in 1748 they were not printed until 1778. Furthermore, the surgeons did not occupy their new Surgeons' Hall at the Old Bailey until 1752. The teaching of anatomy in the new Company did not flourish, even though Pott and William Hunter were elected as first masters of anatomy in 1753. This was due to the excellence of the private schools and many of the best teachers, including John Hunter, preferred to pay the necessary fines rather than teach anatomy in the Surgeons' Company Hall. The appointment of a professor of anatomy in 1760 and professor of surgery in 1790, did not improve matters or the status of the Company. The control of the Company gradually passed into the hands of the ten members of the court of assistants, who were the examiners, and as they were life appointments, old gentlemen in their nineties continued to examine. Little wonder that Astley Cooper protested that "when a man is too old to study, he is too old to be an examiner". The London Company of Surgeons became nothing more than an examining body, satisfied that as long as examinations were carried out, teaching could look after itself, and apprentices were compelled to seek their own teachers. Gunning, the Master of the Company in 1789, strongly criticised the affairs of the Company—"Your theatre is without lecturers, your library without books, and is now an office for your clerk, and your committee room his parlour." The London Company of Surgeons lost their Surgeons' Hall in 1792 and they themselves ceased to have any power after 1797. The College of Surgeons in London received its Royal Charter in 1800 and became the Royal College of Surgeons of England in their new charter of 1843, in which the senior diploma of fellow was introduced.

It is not surprising that the older Royal College of Surgeons in Ireland (1784) with its flourishing Surgeons' School, described as "the most enlightened surgical corporation in Europe", should now run into difficulties with its younger sister College in London. In Dublin the candidate, before becoming a registered pupil in the Surgeons' School, had to pass an examination in Sallust, six books of the Aeneid of Virgil, the Satires and Epistles of Horace, the Greek Testament, Murphy's Lucian, and five books of Homer's Iliad. The registered pupil had to serve apprenticeship for five years and then pass the licence examination of the College. In the Edinburgh and London Colleges there was no such limitation on duration of apprenticeship, and as far as a liberal education was concerned in these Colleges, the candiate could be illiterate and indeed often was. Furthermore, the London College, for its diploma, only required certificates of two courses of anatomy and surgery, which could be taken in one year, and certificates of attendance at a hospital for one year. In 1816 and again in 1818 the Dublin College protested against a bill in the House of Commons, whose provisions would permit diplomates of the London, Edinburgh and Dublin Colleges of Surgeons to practice in any part of the United Kingdom. The Dublin College in their objection stated that they did not wish to be placed in the position of the other Colleges, but on the contrary decreed that all candidates for surgical qualifications should be obliged to study their profession during a reasonably long period. Colles, the occupant of the two College chairs, was the guiding hand in all matters pertaining to the College curriculum, and he always insisted that surgery could only advance in the properly educated and trained man. At this period and for a quarter of a century later, the lowest types of Irish students sought the London diploma. Sir Astley Cooper relates the following anecdote of an Irish candidate before the Examining Board of the London College. "What is a simple fracture and what is a compound fracture?", asked the examiner. The reply was, "A simple fracture is where the bone is broke, and a compound fracture is when it is all broke." Sir Astley asked what he meant by "all broke". "I

mean", he replied, "broken into smithereens to be sure." I
ventured to ask him what was "smithereens". He turned upon
me with an intense expression of sympathy upon his countenance—"You don't know what is 'smithereens'—then I give you
up."

Colles spent long hours in the dissecting room, revising his
anatomical knowledge and planning surgical operations. On
one occasion a student induced the porter of the Surgeons'
School to lend him a key by which he could gain early admission
to the dissecting room. Before six o'clock one morning he was
startled to see Professor Colles walk into the room. "What are
you doing here, sir?" was the interrogatory. The student
explained the position, whereupon the Professor said, "Well,
you are in luck; I am going to make some dissections of the
subjects on these tables, and you shall be my assistant." Colles
probably acquired this habit of early rising and dissection from
his work with Astley Cooper, who dissected daily and was later
to declare, "If I laid my head on my pillow at night without
having dissected something in the day, I should think I lost the
day."

Colles was once asked by his uncle whether he had ever
passed an idle hour. "I passed *two*", was the answer, "and I
saved my life by it, only last Saturday." That Saturday was the
tragical 23rd July, 1803, the date of Emmet's frantic insurrec-
tion. Colles had visited his mother who was staying at Black-
rock, and as it was his birthday he remained longer than he
wished. When he rode back to town, and entered Thomas
Street, on his return to the hospital, he heard the discharge of
the last shot which dispersed the insurgent rabble. At that time
he wore a yeoman's uniform, and had he returned to Dublin
at the time he desired, he must have been in the thick of the
affray.

In 1827, when the class of anatomy in the Surgeons' School
numbered 254, Colles resigned the anatomy chair, but he retained the chair of surgery till 1836.

It is convenient here to leave the College lecture halls and
follow Colles into the wider world of clinical practice. Perhaps
no aspects of the latter are more fascinating and less under-
standable to us now than the universal practice of bloodletting

and the concepts of fever prevailing at that time. Colles was a convinced advocate of bloodletting and never departed from its practice. In this he was no different from his contemporaries. Any doubts in his mind as to its efficacy would certainly have been removed by the Edinburgh school and especially by the dogmatic teaching of Gregory. In 1797 Colles actually defended his M.D. thesis on *De Venaesectione*. Throughout the ages, bloodletting was a common therapeutic measure, especially in fevers and inflammation, and in practice was the main stock-in-trade of the barber surgeons. So universal was its practice that we read only of those who objected to it. The Greeks, Pythagoras and Erasistratus, were averse to it, and in a later century Madame de Sevigne wrote of Chevalier de Grignon, who was seized with smallpox of the most malignant kind—"The physicians immediately proceeded to their favourite practice of bloodletting, the repetition of which, in consequence of the dreadful aggravation of the symptoms which it produced, the patient endeavoured, but ineffectually, to resist. Having been depleted eleven times, he yielded to the combined attack of the doctors and the disease, and expired, a victim of obstinacy and ignorance." In 1727 Dr. Humphrey Markwell, a Dublin practitioner, published anonymously a little volume condemning the practice of indiscriminative venesection which prevailed in his days, and considers that it would be desirable to render bloodletting in smallpox a penal offence unless when performed under medical direction. In 1821, young John Keats, dying of pulmonary tuberculosis and haemoptyses, was treated by bloodletting on several occasions. In the following year an obituary notice in a Dublin newspaper reads:

"After an illness of ten years duration, during which she was bled upwards of 500 times, Mary, only daughter of William Moore, Esq. of Grimeshill, near Kirby, Lonsdale."

Now let Colles describe the treatment of a lung injury, with haemoptyses (and incidentally he was well aware that the patient died not from the blood loss but from tracheal and bronchial obstruction). "Now, suppose we are called in while the profuse bleeding is coming from the mouth—what are we to do? The very best thing we can do is to make the patient faint and thereby to cause a coagulation of the blood. Whenever blood is poured into the cellular membranes, like that which enters into the composition of the lungs, it always coagulates. Well, we induce the fainting by bleeding, and here the bleeding from the arm must be large in quantity and suddenly drawn. The patient's friends may say, "He has already lost large quantities of blood and is still losing it— Why therefore would you take more blood from him?" But do not be deterred from your purpose by anything that may be said or hinted by those who do not understand your object: there is nothing else to save the patient's life. When you open a vein in one arm, if it does not bleed freely, don't hesitate to open a vein in the other, and you must not be satisfied with a small orifice, for ten ounces of blood taken very suddenly, will cause fainting, but it will take twenty ounces to produce the same effect if taken slowly. You *save* blood and the patient's strength in proportion to the freedom with which the blood flows from the vein. But supposing you succeed in lessening or stopping the flow of blood from the mouth, do you relax your vigilance? No, indeed, for in five or six hours it may break out afresh, and you should be on the spot to repeat your venesection instantly: it may return several times in six, ten or twelve hours, and at each recurrence you must be ready with the lancet, and even at every new fit of difficulty of respiration you will bleed if possible—anything to avert haemorrhage from the lungs."

Bloodletting became universal practice in the treatment of fevers in the early decades of the nineteenth century due to the influence of Brown and Gregory of Edinburgh. John Crampton, writing in 1819 of Dr. Steevens' Hospital, says—"Long before the establishment of the different fever hospitals in Dublin it was the only institution where patients affected with fever could be received. Patients so received were admitted to the general wards, sometimes with disastrous results, as it often happened that a single fever patient admitted into a ward with other patients communicated the contagion to every other patient in the ward; nay, sometimes to the whole house, notwithstanding all the precautions take to prevent the contagion spreading." In the fever epidemic 1800–1803, the hospital admitted many cases, but nothing like the numbers admitted to the House of Industry and the newly established fever hospitals. In the epidemic of 1817–1819 special wards of the hospital were opened for fever patients by Dr. William Harvey, but on Harvey's illness and death in 1819, his assistant John Crampton took over their managment. Crampton employed bleeding much more freely than Harvey had done. A full bleeding of the arm or opening the temporal artery was frequently resorted to, and leeches to the head and abdomen were also freely employed. Crampton believed that shaving of the head and the cold effusion after bleeding rendered the future progress of the fever more tractable, and he said that the nurses used to importune him "to direct these measures of depletion for them, of the utility of which they were persuaded from their own observation and experience". William Stokes, describing the practice of that time, says, "I remember when I was a student of the old Meath Hospital, there was hardly a morning that some twenty or thirty sufferers from acute local disease were not phlebotomised. The floor was running with blood, it was dangerous to cross the prescribing hall for fear of slipping; and the scene continued to be witnessed for many years. The cerebral symptoms of typhus fever were met by opening the temporal artery, or by large applications of leeches to the head; and it sometimes happened that the patient died when the leeches were upon his temple—died surely and almost suddenly. An eminent apothecary in this city assured me that when he was serving his apprenticeship there was hardly a week that he was not summoned to take off a large number of leeches from the dead body." Sir D'Arcy Power records that in 1837 at St. Bartholomew's Hospital, London, no less than 96,300 leeches were used, though the number of intern patients treated in the hospital during the year amounted only to 5,557.

Colles' senior medical colleague at Dr. Steevens' Hospital was William Harvey, who had been physician there since 1779. A graduate in arts of Trinity, he graduated M.D. of Edinburgh University in 1774, and also studied at Leiden. Although Physician-General and president of the Physicians' College on some seven occasions, he left little mark on the history of the hospital or in medicine. He appears to have appointed John Crampton as his assistant in 1800, but this appears to have been more of a personal than a hospital appointment, as Crampton was not officially appointed physician until after Harvey's death in 1819. Crampton was more contemporary with Colles and, like him, was a graduate in arts of Trinity in 1789 and M.D. of Edinburgh in 1793. It was no doubt due to the influence of Gregory's teaching in Edinburgh that Crampton showed a greater fondness for the use of the lancet in the treatment of his fever patients than had his predecessor Harvey. Gregory looked on the abstraction of from twelve to twenty ounces of blood as an ordinary bleeding. Quantities under twelve ounces were small and over twenty were large bleedings. Such bleedings were repeated frequently during the course of a fever, and Gregory reports the case of a young man of small stature, who had pneumonia, who in the course of two days and a half lost ninety-eight ounces of blood. The use of alcohol in the treatment of fever patients was then coming into fashion, but the practice did not reach its zenith until some years later, when Dr. Todd recommended that even young patients should get from 36 to 48 ounces of brandy in the twenty-four hours, and that this quantity might be continued over a period of some weeks. One girl of eighteen years of age in an illness of six weeks duration is alleged to have consumed four-and-a-half gallons of brandy.

John Crampton gave lectures in medicine in Dr. Steevens' Hospital for the School of Physic students during the years 1801 to 1804, and again after 1805, pending the building of Sir Patrick Dun's Hospital, but he does not appear to have been a great success as a lecturer in the hospital or as King's professor of materia medica, to which appointment he succeeded in 1804. "Eblanensis" wrote of him . . . "He goes through the business of lecturing like one who is bound to the performance of a heavy task; in fact like some unhappy being who moves round and round in a treadmill for five and twenty long years; while the comparison is rendered still more strikingly applicable by the almost unrecognisable progress he has made. All the allurements of novelty, and of recent interest, are absent from these lectures; and well may his pupils be indifferent to the subject and so

anxious as himself that their short hour should be at an end,
when the professor takes no little pains to conceal his anxiety to
get rid of the business with all convenient speed." Henry
Marsh, who was Crampton's first cousin, became his assistant
in 1820 and physician to Dr. Steevens' Hospital after Crampton's death in 1840. Marsh was then one of the leading physicians in Ireland, and professor of medicine in the Surgeons'
School (1828–1832). He was appointed Physician-in-Ordinary
to the Queen in Ireland in 1837 and received a baronetcy in
1839. Marsh was a colleague, friend and also personal doctor
to Abraham Colles.

In 1833 there were 202 beds available in Dr. Steevens'
Hospital, but they were unequally divided, as there were 172
surgical beds, shared by Colles, Wilmot and Cusack, and about
25 medical beds under the care of Crampton and Marsh.
The clinical teaching in the hospital seems to have been entirely
surgical, there being no arrangement for the clinical teaching of
medicine. With this high complement of surgical beds in the
hospital, and also the growing prestige of Cusack, the resident
surgeon, it was decided to elevate the latter to a new post of
third assistant surgeon, and to fill the vacancy William Colles
was appointed resident surgeon. This appointment of the professor's son to the staff of Dr. Steevens' Hospital did not escape
the attention of Wakley, the "Battling Surgeon" of *The Lancet*,
who devoted an editorial to yet another charge of nepotism.
This "chubby-headed élevè", "the little Lama" as William was
therein called—was later to become Surgeon to the Queen in
Ireland, Regius Professor of Surgery in the University of
Dublin, and President of the Royal College of Surgeons in
Ireland.

In that age, before anaesthesia and antisepsis, the surgeon
who stood at the head of his profession, whether he were a
Guillaume Dupuytren in Paris, an Astley Cooper in London,
or an Abraham Colles in Dublin, was in the popular estimate
little better than a butcher, an object of terror to the shrinking
wretch doomed to suffer his ministrations, and not infrquently a
source of bewilderment and uncertainty to himself. Even
Dupuytren, the "Brigand of Hotel Dieu", master surgeon of
them all, regarded an operation as an "evil alternative, which

nothing short of positive necessity should induce the surgeon to adopt". In the absence of anaesthesia these men had developed a manual dexterity "swift as the sword in the juggler's hand", but the need for sheer speed in the amputation of a limb or the extraction of a bladder stone must often have produced the most unphysiological results. Colles and his Steevens' colleagues do not appear to have performed those rapid "stop-watch" operations which were a feature of the practice of Syme, Liston and others. Steevens' had to wait a few more decades for a "surgical sprinter" in Robert McDonnell, of whom it was said "that if one winked in the theatre while he was cutting for stone, one missed the greater part of the operation". The forte of these Dublin surgeons was their knowledge of surgical anatomy, which by the testimony of Sir Benjamin Brodie was "far ahead of that taught at that time in London or elsewhere". Their surgery was thus a mechanical art, based entirely on their knowledge of anatomy as applied to their art; its science, based on physiological concepts, was yet to be born. The principles on which they based their surgical treatment were derived from the accumulated experience of individuals through the centuries that had gone before. They knew and appreciated the necessity for free drainage of wounds, and that no foreign body, ligature or blood clot, was to remain in the wound. They realised fully that the peritoneum, pleura and dura, so long as they were left intact, could be relied upon as barriers to resist infection from without. But of the reason for the presence of such an infection they had no idea, and the healing *per primum*, so often mentioned in their case reports, bore a looser interpretation than would satisfy any but the indifferent operator today. Suppuration in wounds was acceptable as inevitable; surgeons having long forgotten Theodoric of Lucca and his advocacy of the "dry" treatment of wounds in terms which might have been enunciated by Lister himself:

"It is not necessary, as modern surgeons profess, that pus should be generated in wounds. No error is more grievous than this. Such a practice is indeed to hinder nature, to prolong the disease and to prevent the consolidation of the wound."

This was written in 1266, yet the advocates of "laudable pus" were to have it their own way for six centuries to follow! *In stoliditate sua permittuntur errare** was Theodoric's charitable comment on their obduracy.

None of these Dublin surgeons knew what a micro-organism or leucocyte was, and few were interested in that new toy, the microscope, which John Houston (of the rectal valves), was now introducing into the Dublin medical scene. The scope of their practice was limited. They treated traumatic injuries, wounds, fractures, dislocations and broken skulls, they tapped for dropsy and for hydrocele, they removed superficial tumours with scanty knowledge of their nature, they applied strong nitric acid to piles. The "capital" operations—those which bore the most immediate risk of fatality, included the release of the strangulated hernia, the major amputations, the ligature of the larger arteries for aneurysm, and of course lithotomy. To the surgeon in every hospital was allotted the care of "the venereal", and up to the time of Richard Bright's recognition of nephritis (1827) each and every discomfort associated with the act of urination. The use of the trephine was a "capital operation". Forgetting Ambrose Paré's successful operation at the seige of Metz, Desault (d. 1795) in Paris had declared its employment indefensible, although two of his Irish contemporaries, William Dease (d. 1798) and Sylvester O'Halloran (d. 1807), clearly appreciated that in certain cases of head injury the patient's sole chance of survival might lie in its application. Colles was very conservative in the use of the trephine, warning his students that "the depressed fracture will often recover, although epilepsy may be the consequence later". His contemporary, Cusack Roney, of the Meath Hospital, however, appears to have been more active in the employment of this instrument, when he tells us "that it was by no means unusual in his time when an extern patient presented himself to get a wound in his head dressed, and that it was discovered that a fracture existed, for the surgeon to send him home to his lodgings, and at the same time give directions to the hospital porter to follow him, when the hurry of the morning visit was over, and shave his head and *scalp* him, and that he would call himself either in the

* We allow them their mistake because of their stupidity.

course of the day or the next to trepan him. The hospital porter was in the constant habit of acting as a sort of pioneer to the surgeon, for shaving the head and completely removing an oval piece of the scalp in order to make room for the crown of the trepan." Contemporary accounts of these operations on conscious patients seated upright in a chair read—"it was a dreadful ordeal, cruel and fearful to behold" and "in general if the patient be not unruly, two assistants will suffice." Patients for all operations were drowsed with laudanum or alcohol and strapped down.

Much of Colles' practice would today be considered within the province of the physician and many of his large complement of hospital beds were occupied by cases essentially "medical". He felt equally qualified with the physicians to treat these, especially when William Harvey and John Crampton, the physicians at that time, were not particularly distinguished or even constant in their attendance at the hospital. In this, Colles was no different from Astley Cooper, a great proportion of whose practice was "medical" and who was to write—"Give me opium, tartarised antimony, sulphate of magnesium, calomel and bark, and I would ask for little else."

In 1836 Colles resigned the chair of surgery at the Surgeons' School and was succeeded by William Henry Porter (of the sign). Shortly after this he was presented with the following address by the College—

"Sir . . . in compliance with the unanimous resolution of the Members of the Royal College of Surgeons in Ireland, in College assembled, we wait upon you to express our sincere regret that the pressure of your other professional avocations no longer permit you to discharge the duty of Professor of the Theory and Practice of Surgery in the School of the College. We have also to assure you that it is the unanimous feeling of the College that the exemplary and efficient manner in which you have filled the chair for thirty two years, has been a principal cause of the success and consequent high character of the School of Surgery in this country. It is gratifying to the Members to understand that although they lose the advantage of your valuable services as a Professor in the School of the College, you will still continue to afford your disinterested assistance in promoting the general welfare of the institution, and sustaining the profession of surgery in public estimation. Accept these expressions of our regret for your resignation, and allow us to express our sincere hope that you may long continue to discharge your professional duties with as much advantage to the public as you have to the satisfaction of your professional brethren."

His bust, sculptured by Kirk, and his portrait, painted by Martin Cregan, P.R.H.A., were placed in the College. This portrait was later engraved by Lucas and published in Dublin in 1850.

A handsome piece of silver was also presented to Colles by the College. This was a massive table centre-piece, 30 inches high, weighing 27 pounds, and inscribed:

"Presented by the Royal College of Surgeons in Ireland to Abraham Colles, Esq., in gratitude for services rendered while Professor to the School of Surgery in this country, and in testimony of esteem for professional worth and integrity. Dublin, A.D. 1838."

Near its base are three figures representing the Greek deities Asclepius, Athena, and Hygieia—the same that stand over his College today. Some twenty-five years ago, by a curious lapse of a Colles widow, this family heirloom was presented to the Royal College of Surgeons of England. That College, after enquiries by its president, Webb-Johnson, generously returned the gift to the lineal descendant of Abraham Colles and it is now in the possession of Ronald M. Colles.

In 1839 the growing agitation of medical reform, led by Carmichael and Jacob, proposed a single faculty granting a licence or degree for all Dublin medical practitioners. This proposal was considered at a special meeting of the Royal College of Surgeons in Ireland, and Colles speaking against it, made these remarks—"As to the establishment of one school and licensing body, that would blast the profession. Let there be competition, only for competition with the College of Physicians our scientific meetings would never have been established. Going on with this project is only plunging into a sea of difficulties. It is embroiling us with the other corporations, it will bring down the University upon us, and let it be recollected that the University can grant degrees in surgery. Let us not provoke them to do this—it would be the more valuable degree. . . . Let us labour, every man in his place, to deserve the public confidence, and we must be supported. Let us give up parliamentary business and make a new effort in science. Let the hospital surgeons work the hospitals, and let us all show the advantages of Dublin as a medical school, its University, its cheapness. It had been said that steam would take our pupils and business away from us, but steam went both ways, and the carriages might come here. We ought to bring men here from England to graduate in Trinity College, to study at the Lying-In Hospital. Let us, instead of quarrelling, put forward our advantages and the steamboats would arrive, loaded with English money. Let us only raise the character of our diploma to its former rank—Let us only be united."

Colles, although a professor in a rival medical school always retained his affection for his old University. He went back to Trinity in 1832 for his M.A. degree, and his five sons also graduated there.

In 1850, seven years after Colles' death, the Surgeons' College forgot his advice and provoked the University by refusing to accept its certificates in surgery for its licence. This led Trinity to institute its own licence in surgery in 1851, a M.Ch. degree in 1858, and a B.Ch. degree in 1872—the first University to grant degrees in surgery. Cambridge followed with the degree of master of surgery in 1860/61, and the degree of bachelor of surgery in 1883.

In June 1841 a largely attended meeting of the medical profession was held in Dublin to consider the best means of ensuring the return of a medical member of parliament to represent the interests of the profession. Abraham Colles was called to the chair and there is little doubt that he would have been the representative of the medical profession of Ireland in the Imperial Parliament had the government accepted the principle of professional representation.

In 1841 Abraham Colles resigned as surgeon to Dr. Steevens' Hospital, and his son, William, was appointed his successor. He also ceased to be a governor of the hospital, to which post he had been elected in 1819. During his surgical career, Colles was consultant surgeon to the Lying-in Hospital (Rotunda), the Royal City of Dublin Hospital, the Victoria Lying-in Hospital, and the Pitt Street Institution for Diseases of Children.

CHAPTER 5

Dr. Steevens' Hospital

Man and institutions are formed
by the age to which they belong.
                    Constantia Maxwell, 1946.

At the beginning of the eighteenth century there were only
a few institutions providing for the sick poor. In England only
the monastic houses of St. Bartholomew and St. Thomas
survived the depredations of Henry VIII, although the monasteries associated with them were destroyed. These, with the
House of St. Mary of Bethlehem or "Bedlam" and the small
mineral water hospital at Bath, were the only institutions in
existence. Widdess tells us that prior to the dissolution of the
monasteries, Dublin had four hospitals. The oldest was a twelfth
century foundation attached to the prior of St. John the Baptist,
just without the walls near the New Gate. There were also the
Steyne Hospital on the south bank of the Liffey, founded in
1220 by Archbishop de Loundres, the Hospital of St. Stephen
for lepers, which stood on the site of the present Mercer's
Hospital, and Allen's Hospital in Kevin Street, endowed in
1504 by John Allen, Dean of St. Patrick's, for the sick poor.
At the dissolution, these hospitals were closed and their endow-
ments sold to private individuals. As the eighteenth century
dawned, Dublin had no hospital for its sick poor, although there
was one for its military garrison. It is to the credit of Dublin
that the voluntary hospital system had its inception there, leading to the rapid development of similar institutions throughout
the British Isles, which in themselves provide a wonderful
chapter in the history of medicine. Many of these hospitals
were founded by medical men. The great voluntary hospital
system began in 1718 when six Dublin surgeons founded a
Charitable Infirmary in Cook Street, later transferring to larger

premises in Inn's Quay, and finally to its present site in Jervis Street. Dr. Steevens' Hospital can claim to be the oldest voluntary hospital in so far as it was the oldest in conception and, even more important, it is on the same site, practically in the same fabric, and serving the same function for which it was founded over two-and-a-half centuries ago. As it is justly regarded as the home of Irish surgery, and as it was also the professional home of Abraham Colles for some fifty years, we must take a glance at its history.

Its story begins with one, Reverend John Steevens, a Church of England clergyman of Wiltshire, who encountering Cromwell's displeasure had to flee his cure and his country. It was a strange paradox of history that an Englishman had to emigrate to Ireland to escape Cromwell. At any rate he was now able to see at first hand the results, in terms of destruction and hatred, of that dictator's recent visit to Ireland. Rev. Steevens arrived in Ireland with his wife and twin children, Richard and Grizel, and, after the Restoration, was appointed by Charles II Rector of St. Mary's Church, Athlone. That city in those days was an important place, having its own Royal Charter, and was notoriously Protestant, among its inhabitants being many Quakers. Young Richard Steevens was educated in the Latin School of Athlone and at the age of sixteen entered Trinity in 1670, becoming a scholar of the house four years later, graduating B.A. in 1675 and M.A. in 1678. He appears to have been a student of divinity, but on his father's death in 1682 he changed over to medicine and graduated M.D. in 1687. These were difficult and dangerous times to start a medical career in a city where disease and poverty were rampant, and conditions were not improved by the arrival of James II and his troops, who occupied Trinity and made it a prison for the Protestants of the city. Another John Stevens in his Journal at that time tells us, "drunkenness was so easily prosecuted that no liquors were strong or days long enough to satiate over-hardened drunkards, whilst others, not so seasoned, by often sleeps supplied a weakness of their brain. The women were so suitable to the time that they rather enticed men to lewdness, than carried the least form of modesty, in so much that every quarter of the town might be said to be a public stew. In fine, Dublin seems to be a seminary of vice, an academy of luxury, rather a sink of corruption and a living emblem of Sodom." Conditions were no better in the opposite camp of Schomberg at Dundalk. Out of a total of 14,000 men under that general's command, some 6,300 died of disease.

We know little of the medical practice of Richard Steevens. He did not publish any book on medicine, but nevertheless his standing as a physician must be high, as he was nominated one of the 14 original fellows of the King's and Queen's College of Physicians in their new charter of 1692. In 1703 he was elected president of that College, and was again its president in 1710, in which year he was also appointed professor of Physic at Trinity. In the same year he died, aged 56, unmarried, and left assets of about £12,000. A day or two before he died he asked his twin sister Grizel, whether she had any intention of marrying, and receiving her assurance that she had not, he drew up his will, bequeathing legacies to various friends and to the poor, and his real estate to trustees for the use of his sister during her lifetime, and after her death "to provide one proper place or building within the city of Dublin for a hospital for maintaining and curing from time to time such sick and wounded persons whose distempers and wounds are curable." He died next day and as directed in his will was buried privately and late at night. Dr. Steevens' will made its long and leisurely journey through the high and honourable Court of Chancery and emerged as legal in 1713, but even before that date Madam Steevens, as she was now called, now middle-aged, decided that her brother's wishes should be carried out in her lifetime and in this she had the support of the trustees, prominent amongst whom was Thomas Proby, the Chirurgeon-General. Correspondence with the Duke of Ormonde, the Lord Lieutenant at the time, followed, in an endeavour to influence Queen Anne to get a site and patronage for the project. These efforts ended with the Queen's death in 1714, but Madam Steevens was not deflected from her purpose and she added to the original trustees a group of influential people. These trustees met in 1717 under the chairmanship of William King, Archbishop of Dublin, and announced the purchase of a three-acre site on the south bank of the Liffey within the city boundaries. Captain Thomas

Burgh, Chief Engineer and Surveyor-General of H.M. Fortifica-
tions, was appointed architect. Burgh was architect of many
public buildings at that period and perhaps the greatest production of his art is the magnificent library of Trinity, then in the
course of erection. The hospital building at last got under way
in 1720, but progress was slow and no patients appear to have
been admitted before 1733. Burgh died in 1730 and the hospital
was completed by Pearce. "As a building the hospital may be
called the last kick of the seventeenth century, reproducing on a
smaller scale (115 ft. × 95 ft.) the courtyard and piazza plan
of Robinson's adjacent Royal Hospital. All the detail is cruder
and less sophisticated, making its effect more by quaintness
than by strictly architectural means." (Craig) There is also
some similarity between the design of the hospital and that of
the library of Trinity; both buildings had an open colonnade
on the ground floor and in both the original low roof was in
later times replaced by one of the Mansard type. The very
agreeable little clock tower, with its conoidal hat, was not added
until 1735–6. Early eighteenth-century prints show the hospital
in open ground above the river. Now its closeness to the narrow
Steevens' Lane and the ugly red brick nurses' home between it
and Kingsbridge Station does not show the hospital to advantage
and destroys the scale of the ensemble. In 1720, at the request
of Madam Steevens, Dean Swift was appointed an additional
trustee and remained a member of its board until his death in
1745. With the death of the important trustees—King in 1729,
Proby in 1729, and Burgh in 1730—it was necessary to have an
act of the Irish Parliament passed in 1730 to safeguard the future
of the hospital. This act constituted a new board of governors
consisting of the highest dignitaries of the Church and State.

Thomas Proby, a personal friend of Dr. Steevens and a trustee
named in his will, was then the leading surgeon in Ireland.
Born in Dublin in 1665 and qualified by apprenticeship, he
was present at a dissection of a malefactor at the College of
Physicians in 1672, and was appointed Chirurgeon-General in
Ireland in 1699. In 1694 he operated on Dorcas Blake, a young
woman of twenty, and removed a 4 inch ivory bodkin from her
urinary bladder. This woman made an excellent recovery, but
the nature of the operation created a sensation in Dublin at

that time. Dragged before the Lord Mayor by the news hawks of the day, she made oath and swore "that the above relation is true in substance and that she had swallowed the bodkin therein mentioned"—a perfectly reasonable answer by any young woman in such a predicament. Proby's operation by the high route is probably the first recorded example of supra-pubic cystotomy and details of the case were communicated to the Royal Society and published in its *Transactions* in 1710 by Sir Thomas Molyneux, who was present at the operation. Proby was a skilful operator and took an active interest in improving the professional standards of the Barber Surgeons, though as an Army surgeon he was not a member of their guild. Between 1703 and 1713 he was in frequent communication with the Physicians about the promotion of a bill in parliament to regulate the practice of surgery. Proby and his wife were close friends of Swift and Esther Johnson and he is frequently mentioned by Swift in *The Journal to Stella*. Proby in later life was saddened by the behaviour of his eldest son, Captain Proby, "who dis-covered an inclination to Popery while he was quartered with his regiment in Galway". The captain was courtmartialled and resigned his commission. He subsequently received one shilling in his father's will. In that will Proby directed that his chirurgical instruments be given to Dr. Steevens' Hospital and that he be buried in the chapel, in a strong oak coffin, not covered, with the "date of my age and death studded with small neat nails on top of it", and further directed that his son-in-law, John Nicols, who succeeded him as Chirugeon-General, should before his burial cut off the big toe of his left foot and part of the adjoining metatarsus and preserve it for observation how to prevent or cure the like disorder in other persons who have had the misfortune to be afflicted with it.

Jonathan Swift, the great Dean of St. Patrick's Cathedral, requires no introduction to the reader. He was appointed a trustee of Dr. Steevens' Hospital in 1720, and although never very active in the management of the hospital, his influence has been felt throughout its whole history. The success of Dr. Steevens' Hospital no doubt influenced the Dean in his decision to endow a hospital when as far back as 1731 he wrote his brilliantly cynical *Verses on the Death of Dr. Swift*.

"He gave the little wealth he had
To build a house for fools and mad,
And showed by one satyric touch
No nation wanted it so much."

In his last will dated 1740 he directed his trustees to dispose of his fortune "by purchasing lands of inheritance situated in any province in Ireland except Connaught and from the yearly profits of these to purchase a piece of land situated near Dr. Steevens' Hospital and to build a hospital there large enough for the reception of as many idiots and lunatics as the annual increase of the said lands and worldly substance will be sufficient to maintain, and I direct that the said hospital be called St. Patrick's Hospital". Swift died in 1745 and humanity, as well as Ireland, has much to learn from his own famous epitaph in Latin in the walls of his cathedral.

"Here lies the body of Jonathan Swift
    of this cathedral church, Dean
Where savage indignation cannot lacerate
    his heart any more.
Traveller go, and imitate if you can
His strenuous vindication of man's liberty."

In 1746 Swift's trustees were appointed Governors of St. Patrick's Hospital by Royal Charter of George II. The governors of Dr. Steevens' Hospital, when approached, willingly gave up part of their ground for the creation of St. Patrick's Hospital (often referred to as Swift's Hospital) which was completed in 1757. Ever since then the two great institutions have worked side by side for the relief of those disordered in body and mind. When Esther Johnson, "Stella", died she bequeathed £1,000 to Dr. Steevens' Hospital for the maintenance of a chaplain, a request no doubt due to her friendship with Proby.

One of the treasures of the hospital is the Worth library. Dr. Edward Worth was a cultured physician in the city in the first thirty years of the eighteenth century, and was one of the extra trustees appointed to the hospital by Madam Steevens. He was a true bibliophile and his collection of some four thousand volumes on medicine and general subjects with magnificent bindings are still displayed in their original cases.

The Dr. Steevens' Hospital Act of 1730 constituted a new board of governors; the most important of these was the Primate, Hugh Boulter. He was an active governor of the hospital from 1730 till his death in 1742. He fitted up a ward at the hospital, of ten beds, at his own expense in 1736, and this has since been known as the "Lord Primate's Ward". He was a warm friend of the hospital and one of the most influential men in Ireland, but by his devotion to the English interest made many enemies among those with whom he lived. On one occasion he complained that if an Englishman were not appointed to the vacant see of Cashel there would be "thirteen Irish to nine English bishops which we think would be a dangerous situation". Neither his conduct as a politician nor his position as a theologian concerns us here; of his charity there can be no question. He took a particular interest in the welfare of the hospital, and presided frequently at its governors' meetings. He supported five beds, in addition to fitting up a ward at his own expense. As an Englishman, it is only fitting that the monument to his memory was placed in Westminster Abbey:

"He was born January 4, 1671,
He was consecrated Bishop of Bristol 1718,
He was translated to the Archbishopric
    of Armagh 1723
And from thence to Heaven."

The hospital received its patients about 1733 and shortly after this Owen Lewis was elected the second or resident surgeon. Two years later, however, he was dismissed at the request of Madam Steevens, and was replaced by Samuel Butler. In 1740 John Nicols, the Surgeon-General, gave the hospital £805 5s. 6d., being the proceeds of a third share of a lottery—the Charitable Infirmary of Inns Quay, and Mercer's Hospital being the other beneficiaries. Apart from this lottery, Dr. Steevens' Hospital never again took part in one, although for Bartholomew Mosse's Lying-in Hospital, lottery funds were very much employed for its erection and maintenance.

In the early part of the eighteenth century the teaching of medicine in western Europe was dominated by Hermann Boerhaave. As professor of medicine, botany and chemistry in the University of Leiden, Boerhaave attracted students from all over the world, and among them were very many men from Ireland who on their return home spread the doctrines of their teacher. Boerhaave, the most learned physician of his day, was called the "Batavian Hippocrates" or the "Modern Galen" and though he had little title to the rank of Hippocrates, yet his influence on the medical teaching of his time was enormous. His *Institutions* (1708) and his *Aphorisms* (1709) were translated into many languages, and were studied throughout the world; yet in spite of his great reputation he added little of permanent value to our knowledge. He was the most brilliant exponent of the "blind alley", but his brilliance retarded rather than encouraged those who might have sought the true path. Sir Clifford Albutt said of him that he "seems to have contented himself with hashing up the partial truths and entire errors of his time". In reality, as is often the case with teachers, his influence was due to his personality more than to his knowledge, and to the lucid forcible way he taught his views, rather than to the actual value of those views. The influence of Boerhaave's teaching lasted for a considerable time after his death, especially in France, but it was nothing like so great as it had been during his lifetime. His pupils carried away with them the forms and system of their master, but not his personality. Those of them like von Haller, Monro, Whytt, Albinus, Cullen and Barry, who rose to eminence in the profession, made many advances in our knowledge, but they made these advances not so much by maintaining the system of their master, as by new discoveries and observations. Lindeboom in a recent biography places Boerhaave in a more favourable light, especially his experimental work in chemistry and his great publication, *Elementa Chemiae*. This biographer points out that the *Institutions* and *Aphorisms* did not represent Boerhaave's lectures, but rather headings for his lectures to his students; Lindeboom also stresses Boerhaave's influence on the development of three great universities—Edinburgh, through Monro and his associates; Gottingen through von Haller; and Vienna through Van Swieten; all students at Leiden. Underwood, also, has recently emphasised Boerhaave's greatness.

Little information has come down to us of the medical and surgical practice of the hospital during its early years, nor do we know much of the life and work of the different members of the staff. It is doubtful if Grattan, Helsham and Robinson, the first physicians of the hospital, were ever pupils of Boerhaave. James Grattan, a King's professor of medicine, probably never lectured in Trinity as there were few students; and there was no salary, as Lady Dun was still alive. Richard Helsham was professor of natural philosophy or mathematical physics as well as professor of medicine. He was a member of the Swift circle and appears to have acted as physician to the great Dean. In a letter to Pope in 1728 Swift describes his physician thus. "Here is an ingenious, good-humoured physician, a fine gentleman, an excellent scholar, easy in his fortunes, kind to everybody, hath abundance of friends, entertains them often and liberally, they pass the evening with him at cards, with plenty of good meat and wine, eight or a dozen together; he loves them all and they him, he hath twenty of them at command, if one of them dies, he is no more than poor Tom! He getteth another, or taketh up with the rest and is no more moved than at the loss of his cat; he offended nobody, is easy with everybody—is not this the true happy man?" Helsham died in 1738, and in a codicil to his will, he wrote "as to my funeral, it is my wish (and I do adjure my executors not to fail in the execution of it) that before my coffin be nailed up my head be severed from my body and that my corpse be carried to the place of burial by the light of one taper only, at the dead of night, without hearse or pomp attended by my domesticks only". Helsham's lectures in natural philosophy were published in 1739 by his friend and pupil, Bryan Robinson, being the first scientific work printed at the University press. Many subsequent editions of his book were issued and it continued to be used as a text-book in the University for nearly a hundred years.

Bryan Robinson, a leading physician of his day, acted as physician to the hospital in 1733, 1737 and 1741. He was formerly lecturer in anatomy at Trinity and later Regius professor of Physic. In addition to editing Helsham's lectures, he published a famous text-book, the *Animal Economy*, in 1732. He was an ardent admirer of Sir Isaac Newton and endeavoured to account for animal motions and even the rational treatment of disease on Newtonian principles. His chapter on respiration is a remarkable one. He speaks in it of a certain portion of the air, which he calls the acid part, mixing with the blood in the lungs and being essential to life. Oxygen was not discovered until thirty-one years after the appearance of Robinson's work, and it is interesting to note that Lavoisier, who gave to oxygen its name, believed it to be the former of acids. Like others, Robinson spent his energies in building up a system of medicine founded on a very imperfect knowledge of the functions of the body, and though the system was fortified by careful mathematical reasoning it soon disappeared as advancing knowledge altered fundamentally the concepts to which that reasoning applied. It is interesting to note that Abraham Colles attended a course of lectures on the Animal Economy by J. Allery in Edinburgh in 1796.

Henry Cope, the State Physician, also acted as physician to the hospital in 1734. He was Regius professor of Physic in Trinity and enjoyed an extensive practice in the city. Shortly after, he had some domestic trouble referred to by Swift in a letter to Sheridan in 1735. "Here have been five and forty devils to do about Dr. Cope's daughter, who ran away with a rogue, one Gibson, and the doctor caught them in a field with a hedge parson in the act of coupling." Sheridan replied "Dr. Cope was a fool to trouble himself about his rampant daughter; for he may be assured though he secures her from the present lover, since the love fit is upon her she will try either his butler or his coachman." Henry Cope's granddaughter Sophia Cope was cast in a different mould; she became the wife of Abraham Colles. The Cope family pedigree (see Appendix) is not only distinguished but also of some historical interest. It stems from Sir Anthony Cope, Vice-Chamberlain to Catherine Parr (1512–1548), sixth wife of Henry VIII. Catherine, like her Royal spouse was not designed to live alone, and five weeks after the King's death in 1547, she married Lord Seymour—her fourth husband.

Clinical practice in the early days of the hospital was very different from what prevails at the present time. In 1733 when the hospital was opened the governors defined precisely the duty of each officer and servant. The physician was to visit the sick each Monday and Friday, at 11 o'clock in the morning and oftener if occasion required. At these visits he was to give directions to the second surgeon and nurses as he should see proper. The first surgeon was to visit at the same hours with the physician, to perform all chirurgical operations, and to give such directions in surgical cases as he should see proper. The second, or resident surgeon, was to act also as apothecary and was to prepare and keep the medicines. He was to mix and deliver to the nurses the medicines prescribed by the physician and first surgeon, to dress the patients' wounds, to perform such operations in surgery as he should be directed to by the first surgeon, and to reside constantly in the house. The most important duty of the physician and first surgeon when they attended on Monday and Friday was to examine the persons who applied to be admitted as patients into the hospital. This examination took place in the committee room, not in the wards. It was only occasionally that it was considered necessary for the physician to visit the wards, as he prescribed for the patients on their admission and the subsequent care of them was entrusted to the second or resident surgeon. At a time when physicians learned their practice entirely from books, when they explained disease by *a priori* reasoning, and founded their practice on such explanations, minute and frequent examination of the patient was not of much consequence and was indeed rather beneath the dignity of the great man. Till much later in the century many physicians in practice never saw large numbers of the patients they prescribed for, but relied entirely on the report of the cases submitted by the attending apothecary or surgeon. Physicians like Radcliffe and Mead, who held high positions as consultants in London, were in the habit of meeting surgeons and apothecaries in some coffee-house, and then giving their opinion and directions for the treatment of the patients whose cases were submitted to them. Boerhaave did an extensive consultation practice by letter, as did Cullen of Edinburgh till the time of his death in 1790.

The "surgeon's patients" were treated in the same wards as

the "doctor's patients" and were about equally divided in numbers. In 1750 some sixty-six patients were in residence in the hospital. The chirurgical operations were performed by the surgeons in the room called the "surgery", there being no special room set apart as an operating theatre. John Nicols who succeeded his father-in-law, Thomas Proby, as Surgeon-General in 1728 acted as first surgeon to the hospital for twenty-three years, and later became a visiting surgeon. He is reported as having been a skilful operator, but we do not know anything of the work of the other two surgeons. In 1735 Nicols cut a child of five years old for stone, which stone was as large as a pullet's egg and weighed three-quarters of an ounce. It was stated that "the child had a good appetite and is likely to do well". In 1757 "a child about seven years old who was previously afflicted with the gravel, had a stone extracted from her, the bigness of an ordinary hen's egg, in Steevens' Hospital and a few months later another member of the same family was cut for stone in the hospital". Many of the surgical patients who were admitted were suffering from the result of accidents and assaults; abscesses and leg ulcers were common, as were cancer of the lip and empyema. One man had "a phagedenic ulcer where his penis used to be". In September 1755 a poor woman, the wife of one Kelly, was tapped for dropsy in Dr. Steevens' Hospital and a large quantity of water extracted. What is pretty remarkable was that next day she was delivered of a child, though she herself was utterly ignorant of her pregnancy.

At the time patients were first admitted to the hospital, Madam Steevens was no longer a young woman, being in her seventy-eighth year. We do not know when she first took up residence in the hospital, but she probably did so some years before it opened for patients in 1733. She lived in rooms on the ground floor just to the south side of the entrance gate. Probably she kept a general supervision over the management of the hospital, but there is not any evidence of interference by her with the duties of the resident officers. Her action in connection with Owen Lewis, the first resident surgeon, is the sole recorded instance of her making any suggestions as to either the officers or their work. The minutes of the board meetings and the papers preserved in the hospital are singularly silent regarding her. Regularly, till the time of her death, she paid considerable sums of money to the treasurer for the use of the hospital, but these were received as a matter of course, without any formal acknowledgement in the minutes. In 1742 Madam Steevens was allowed to have her faithful servant, Margaret Stevenson, to live with her in the hospital, and in April 1740, being weak and infirm, she signed her will which was witnessed by Richard Butler, the resident surgeon. In this she desired that she should be buried late at night at St. Peter's Church, where her mother and brother were buried before her, and that her funeral should be conducted in "as private a manner as possible". To Margaret Stevenson she gave £200, her silver and household goods, and smaller amounts of money to her friends, including £10 to the Reverend Peter Cooke, the hospital chaplain and also her executor, and finally the residue of her estate to the governors of the hospital for the use of the said hospital. She died on the 17th March 1746 in the ninety-third year of her age. There had been a meeting of the governors on March 5th, and two days after Madam Steevens died they met again. At this meeting the Primate was in the chair, the Archbishop of Dublin, the Bishop of Elphin, the Dean of St. Patrick's, and eight other members of the board were present. Madam Steevens lay dead in the hospital, but there is no mention of the fact made in the minutes of the meeting, nor is there any record of the governors' appreciation of her work. They decided that when "the balance which shall remain in the hands of Madam Steevens' executors" was paid in, a new ward should be opened in the hospital. Besides this decision, various other items of business were transacted, just as if nothing unusual had occurred. For some reason the executors decided that she should be buried in St. James' Church instead of St. Peter's Church, as desired in the will, and whether it was at night or not we do not know. Ten years later the body of Madam Steevens was transferred to the vault under the chancel of the present chapel. At the time of the last removal the four coffins in the vault were found to be so decayed that it was impossible to be sure which belonged to Madam Steevens, but a small piece of silk ribbon was found to be quite intact and had probably formed part of her shroud.

The governors of the hospital received £225 4s. 11½d. out of her estate of £882 4s. 1d.

It is necessary to refer here to the story about Madam Steevens which gained a wide publicity in Ireland during the nineteenth century. It was stated that she was born with a pig's face, was fed out of a silver trough, and that in consequence of the deformity she was led to devote her life to charity. Some said even that the story was current in her lifetime, owing to her habit of going amongst the poor heavily veiled, when on visits of charity, and that to contradict the story she used to sit at her window in the hospital to allow the people to see her. There is absolutely no evidence of the truth of this story in contemporary records, nor indeed does it appear to have been connected with the good lady until the nineteenth century. The story as then told runs as follows—Just before the birth of Madam Steevens her mother was visited by a poor woman with three children, who asked for bread. While refusing to help her, Mrs. Steevens had told the woman to get away with her litter of pigs. In return for this the woman put a curse on her and her unborn child, with the result that when the child was born it had the face of a pig. At one time the story was widely believed and visitors to the hospital have asked to see the silver trough out of which Madam Steevens used to be fed. Some even went so far as to assert that they had seen the trough in the hospital. It is not known who first associated the story with Madam Steevens, but some of the permanent officers in the early part of the last century were in the habit of telling it to visitors to the hospital. Possibly they derived some pecuniary benefit by showing the supposed trough to the curious, but it is more likely that they told the story as a test of the credulity of their auditors, and possibly by repetition of it came to believe it themselves. This much, however, is certain—there is not a shadow of foundation for the truth of the story as applied to the good Madam Steevens. Actually such stories were current centuries before, and Kirkpatrick makes reference to pamphlets with similar stories published in London in 1640, and in Amsterdam in 1641.

In 1749, Dr. William Stephens was appointed visiting physician to the hospital. It is not known whether he was any

relative of Richard and Grizel Steevens. A graduate of Trinity
and of Leiden, he was president of the Physicians' College in
1733, 1742 and 1759. He appears to have been associated with
the teaching of botany in the early days of the medical school
of Trinity and published a pamphlet of some fifty pages for the
guidance of its medical students. Stephens was in the chair at
a meeting in the rooms of the Philosophical Society in Trinity
in 1731 when the Royal Dublin Society was founded. He was
later a lecturer in chemistry in Trinity and published a book
in London in 1732 upon the cure of gout by milk diet. He died
suddenly at Wexford in 1760 of "gout in the stomach". Kirkpatrick remarks that his portrait in the hospital "does not
suggest that he had treated his gout by strict adherence to a
milk diet"! A few years before his death, William Stephens
invited a young Trinity graduate, Samuel Clossy, to study morbid anatomy and make post-mortem examinations at Dr.
Steevens' Hospital. Clossy later worked at St. George's Hospital,
London, and published a book on morbid anatomy. Later he
was for a short period physician to Mercer's Hospital, Dublin.
Then he emigrated to New York in 1763, and became the first
professor of anatomy at King's College, now Columbia
University.

The original surgical staff of the hospital remained almost
unchanged for some twenty years, but in 1756 it was re-
organised. The visiting surgeons, which included the Surgeon-
General were now to be strictly honorary, and the active
surgical staff was henceforth to consist of two assistant surgeons
and the resident surgeon. John Whiteway and Samuel Croker
were the first assistant surgeons to be appointed. Both had been
apprentices to John Nicols at the hospital and both were later
to attain high rank in their profession. Whiteway was a relative
of Dean Swift, who paid his apprenticeship fees, and in the
Dean's will he received £100 to qualify him as a surgeon. When
the great Dean died in 1745 it was Whiteway who performed
the post-mortem examination. The Dean seems to have anticipated that his body would after death be subjected to close
scrutiny, for in his verses *On the Death of Dr. Swift* (1731) he
writes:

"The doctors, tender of their fame,
Wisely on me lay all the blame.
We must confess his case was nice;
But he would never take advice.
Had he been ruled, for aught appears,
He might have lived those twenty years;
For, when we open'd him, we found
That all his vital parts were sound."

Whiteway opened the skull, but all we now know of the condition of the brain thereby exposed is that it contained "much water". Whiteway, described as "one of the principal surgeons of the city of Dublin", signed the petition to incorporate the Irish College of Surgeons and in the Royal Charter granted in February 1784 he was named as one of the members. In 1786 he was elected the second president of the College. Samuel Croker, who took the additional name of King under the terms of a bequest made to him by Miss Jane King, soon became one of the leading surgeons in Dublin and enjoyed a large and fashionable practice. The Duke of Wellington, as a child, was one of his patients, and Cameron tells us that it was due to Croker-King's treatment that the child's life was saved. Croker-King was nominated as the first president of the Royal College of Surgeons in Ireland, and in 1785 he wrote a short history of Dr. Steevens' Hospital.

The appointment of Whiteway and Croker-King, both young men, as assistant surgeons in 1756, should have placed the hospital in a favourable position for doing good work, but surprisingly they contributed little to its advancement at that time. Philip Woodroffe was appointed assistant surgeon in 1762, but four years later preferred to revert to resident surgeon, a post which at that time and indeed for many years later was considered to be the more important. Woodroffe was to hold office for thirty-three years, but in spite of his long tenure he also left little mark in the history of the hospital. He was, however, a noted surgeon of his day, and had a large private practice and many apprentices. As a member of the Dublin Society of Surgeons, he signed the petition for the charter of the Royal College of Surgeons, in which he was named one of the original members, and was present at the first meeting of the College. Two years later he was elected treasurer of the College, and in 1788 while still resident surgeon was chosen president of the College. In addition to his Steevens' appointment he was surgeon to the Foundling's Hospital, the Hospital for Incurables, and consulting surgeon to the House of Industry. Gilborne refers to him in the following lines—

"Woodroffe redresses all chirurgic woes,
Amputated stumps he covers with Lambeau's;
To make the maimed live out their time with ease
A practice quite unknown in Ancient Days."

It was to Woodroffe that young Colles was apprenticed, and Colles was also to be his successor.

When Abraham Colles, just twenty-six years of age, was appointed resident surgeon to the Steevens' Hospital in July 1799, he had as colleagues on the staff of the hospital, William Harvey who had been physician since 1779; Samuel Croker-King and George Stewart (Surgeon-General), visiting surgeons; Ralph Smith Obre and James Boyton, assistant surgeons. By right of his position Colles had under his personal charge one-third of the surgical beds, and we may feel sure he got more than his share of the surgical work, as Boyton did not attend the hospital regularly.

Immediately on his appointment the governors asked Colles to make a list of the surgical instruments belonging to the hospital, and Kirkpatrick tells us that the list in his hand-writing is still preserved. There was a case of instruments for lithotomy, containing staffs, sounds, gorgets, double-edged scalpels, forceps, and scoops. There were also cases of amputating instruments, two sets of "scarifying and cupping instruments", a case of "trepanning instruments" and a catheter case containing one female and five male catheters. In addition to these there were two sets of dissecting knives, two sets of "tobacco smoke bellows with two tubes", one set of three silver hare lip pins with moveable steel points, and thirty-three single instruments. Some of these instruments may have been those bequeathed to the hospital by Surgeon-General Proby in 1729, and some of those purchased in 1768 by Surgeon-General Ruxton and Mr. Whiteway, at the request of the governors. The list is of interest as it shows what was considered necessary in the *armamentarium chirurgicum* of a large hospital at the beginning of the nineteenth century. Unfortunately none of these instruments can now be identified in the hospital. The bellows for tobacco smoke were used at that time for giving rectal injections of tobacco smoke in order to cause the patient to faint, and so to allow a relaxation of the muscles which would facilitate the reduction of dislocations and of hernia. This crude apparatus for burning tobacco over heated coals and insufflating the smoke by means of the bellows and tube into the rectum produced many uncalled-for and even disastrous results. Colles after many trials abandoned its use and substituted instead the tobacco enema. It is interesting that there is no mention of a tracheostomy tube in the list, and even remarkable when one remembers that William Dease had warmly advocated the operation of bronchotomy in his book *Observations on Wounds of the Head* published in 1778. Dease had had himself performed the operation, though unsuccessfully, and he illustrates two double silver cannulas of different sizes, so that the inside one may be drawn out occasionally and cleaned.

As the eighteenth century closed, with Colles about to begin his career, the hospital was in serious difficulties for funds. Prices of all the necessary commodities were rising rapidly and the disturbed state of the country, following the Rebellion and the Union, did not favour charitable institutions. Already, in 1792, the governors had decided to close two wards, "that a fund may accumulate to a sum sufficient to put the building into complete repair". Then, in 1799, Robert Perceval and George Stewart were asked to report on the whole economy of the house. Perceval was keen on the reduction of the patients' dietary, but this the governors did not agree to. In 1800, the governors decided that "no servant be admitted to Dr. Steevens' Hospital without the sum of two guineas being sent with such servant" by his or her master. This was a legitimate proposal, provided it was not interpreted too strictly. At a meeting of the hospital board in 1800 with Isaac Corry, Chancellor of the Exchequer, and Earl Clare the Lord Chancellor, present; the noble Lords' proposal was "that a petition be forthwith made to Parliament to empower the governors to dispose of the books bequeathed by Edward Worth, to the best advantage for the use of the said hospital". It is little wonder that the affairs of the country were in the state they were when two of its chief executive officers could entertain such a proposal as remedy for the difficulties that confronted the hospital. In 1801 the hospital, through one of its most able governors, Lord Kilwarden, the Lord Chief Justice, petitioned the Imperial Parliament for funds to maintain itself, but Parliament did not at that time make any grant to the hospital and the governors were compelled to sell some of their investments. Lord Kilwarden was subsequently murdered while returning to town in his carriage during the Emmet Rebellion of July 1803. In that year relief came to the hospital from an unexpected quarter. The Army authorities required extra hospital accommodation for the troops of the Dublin garrison and the governors quickly agreed to allot the top floor of the hospital for the use of the troops at a reasonable rental. Though two years was the limit fixed upon, as a matter of fact the military continued in occupation of the premises for eleven years, and many of the soldiers wounded in the Peninsular War were treated in Dr. Steevens' Hospital. They caused singularly little disturbance to the general working of the house, and their tenancy ended in December 1814. Meanwhile Kilwarden's original petition was again placed before Parliament and this time the response was generous, as in the twenty-five years, 1805 to 1829 inclusive, sums amounting to £40,860 16s. 11d. were given to the hospital.

When James William Cusack was appointed resident surgeon in 1813, on terms of appointment similar to his predecessors', the governors at the time adopted a code of rules which defined more precisely the duties of the resident surgeon. They gave into his charge all the surgical instruments belonging to the hospital and made him responsible for their safe-keeping. He was directed to summon the visiting surgeons and the assistant surgeons in all cases where the patient needed a "capital" operation; and he was also to inform them of all operations that were to be performed. This custom persisted in the hospital until recent years, and it was the practice of the whole surgical staff to visit the wards together on certain days in order to consult about the patients. Early hours were to be the rule in the hospital, and the resident surgeon was directed to see that all surgical patients were dressed by eight o'clock in the summer and nine o'clock in the winter, except on visiting days. He was also to visit all the wards each morning to receive a report from the nurse of each, stating every circumstance that might possibly require his speedy attention. The important duty was assigned to him of having a general superintendence of the internal economy of the hospital—a regulation that made him the chief executive officer of the house, and this position the resident surgeon has enjoyed ever since. All patients who were brought into the hospital suffering from accidents were to be under his care, but in cases of difficulty or such as required sudden operation he was to summon the assistant surgeons. Finally, the resident surgeon was now elected for seven years, with eligibility for re-election, but this rule never seems to have applied to Cusack, as he held office without re-election until 1834.

In the early years of its existence, ventilation of the hospital, if at all considered in its construction, seems to have presented no problem. The hospital was sited on open ground, its wards were lofty, its patients few in number. John Wesley, who visited the hospital in 1749, records "I saw Dr. Steevens' Hospital far cleaner and sweeter than any I had seen in London". John Howard, the philanthropist, visited Dublin in 1779 and again several times in later years. In his first report he says, "Many of the hospitals in Dublin may be viewed with pleasure—Steevens', Simpson's, St. Patrick's and the Infirmary of the Foundling Hospital, were some of the cleanest". On subsequent visits he was not so complimentary to Steevens'—"The wards were close and offensive, the windows were shut when the days were fine. The indiscriminate admission of visitants is *highly* improper, especially of men into women's wards, and more particularly when the beds, as here, are enclosed with wood and curtains. I have seen a person come for admission to the hospital when the effects of frequent use of spirituous liquor have appeared by the dropsical water forcing itself through the pores of the skin." Howard also noted "that the sand on the ward floor was well soaked with the spits and accidental dirt occasioned by the patients." Notwithstanding his remarks, we find that sand was used on the ward floors as late as 1787, three years before young Colles arrived as a student. There can be little doubt that it was due to conditions inside rather than outside the hospital that the subject of ventilation attracted so much attention. The surgical wards, overcrowded with septic patients, and the medical wards with those suffering from all kinds of fever, must have made any lack of ventilation very obvious. It is evident, also, that the governors, though anxious for fresh air, knew little about the way of obtaining it, apart from cutting down trees around the hospital and purchasing a copy of the Marquis of Chabane's book (1815) on ventilation. It was not, however, until many years later that the obvious plan of opening large windows from the wards into the corridors was adopted, a plan which has made the wards at the present time as well ventilated as those of any hospital in the city.

In 1820 the governors of Dr. Steevens' Hospital received a letter from the Viceroy requesting accommodation for male patients from the Westmoreland Lock Hospital. This was to have an important influence on the whole subsequent history of the hospital and on the career of Abraham Colles. The Lock Hospital was first opened in Rainsfort Street in 1755 and was said to have been "the first of its kind in the kingdom". In 1778 it was moved to the Buckingham Hospital in Donnybrook, which had been built by the City Corporation as a smallpox hospital, but had never been used for that purpose. The move to the Buckingham Hospital did not prove to be a success; the situation was too remote from the city to attract patients, even had there been funds sufficient to support them. In almost all the city hospitals there was a prejudice against admitting patients with venereal disease, and as there were many such patients the accommodation was wholly inadequate. As a result these patients became a serious burden on the House of Industry, to which most of them drifted. In 1792, as the result of representation to the Government, Lord Westmoreland, the Viceroy, took the matter in hand. At that time the Hospital for Incurables, founded by the Charitable Musical Society on the Blind Quay in 1744 was now located in a large stone house in Lazars' Hill, to which it had been moved in 1755. Lazars' Hill, the site of an old leper hospital—corrupted to "Lousy Hill"—is now known as Townsend Street. The situation of this hospital in the heart of the city was just as unsuitable as the Lock Hospital in the suburbs, and, like the Lock Hospital, the Hospital for Incurables was then in a languishing condition. At the insistence of Lord Westmoreland, an exchange was effected—the Hospital for Incurables went to Donnybrook, and the Lock Hospital was moved from Donnybrook to the house on Lazars' Hill. The accommodation of the latter house was to be increased so as to provide three hundred beds, while the funds for its support were to be supplied by Parliament. In 1792 the new Lock Hospital was opened with one hundred and twenty-eight beds for the indiscriminate admission, without recommendation, of indigent persons with venereal disease. Further beds were added in 1796, when the total reached two hundred and fifty. From 1792 to 1800, 11,386 patients were admitted to the wards of which 10,679 were discharged cured, 242 died, and 237 were discharged for irregular conduct, and 238 remained in the hospital. In addition to these, some 16,934 patients were treated as "externs". Difficulties arose in the management of the hospital, not surprisingly, with this type of patient, but later on the irregularities in the hospital became notorious. The house was overcrowded, and yet only a small proportion of those seeking relief could be admitted. The ventilation was so bad that "a mercurial atmosphere is therefore formed, by which spitting is often prematurely produced, and thus the exhibition of mercury to such an extent, and in such quantity as to afford a probable chance of affecting a radical cure is prevented". Further, rule by restraint, compulsory detention, the presence of a military guard and provision of underground cells for refractory patients, only made matters within the hospital worse, and did not prevent 250 patients from eloping in the space of three years. Reports of further commissions showed that conditions had gone from bad to worse, and eventually they became a public scandal. It was at this stage that the Viceroy decided that the institution should in future be opened for female patients only. In 1820, Dr. Steevens' Hospital agreed to receive thirty of the remaining male patients, and their beds from the Lock Hospital; the former were described as "worn out objects" and the latter as being in "a most abused state". Thus ended the career of the Lock Hospital as a mixed institution. Perhaps the most important benefit that the community derived from the change then effected, and from the opening of the Lock wards at Dr. Steevens' Hospital, was the facility afforded for the instruction of medical students. One of the regulations of the Lock Hospital was that apprentices and students were not on any account to be introduced into the wards, and had it not been for the wards of Dr. Steevens' Hospital there would have been little clinical material in Dublin for teaching students the diagnosis and treatment of this important group of diseases. Two of the empty wards on the top landing of the hospital were opened for the reception of patients from the Lock Hospital, and these wards were kept well supplied with patients. It was largely from the experience gained there that Colles was able to write his treatise, and ever since Dr. Steevens' Hospital has been an important centre for the study of all forms of venereal disease.

Solomon Richards was for a short while visiting surgeon after Croker-King's death in 1817, but was little interested in surgery, having won a lottery prize of £10,000. He was described as "the biggest and fattest surgeon in the United Kingdom". Richards and Obré—described as a very small man, were very close friends. One night when returning from an operation in the country their carriage was stopped by armed robbers, who presented pistols at Richards and demanded his money, relieving him also of his watch and a case of surgical instruments. Obré concealed behind his big friend, quite escaped notice and the carriage was about to proceed on its journey when Richards drew the attention of the robbers to Obré. They at once relieved him also of his valuables. This having been done, Richards suggested to the highwaymen that having got Obré's money through his kindness, his watch and surgical instruments might be returned. The suggestion was agreed to and the pair were allowed to proceed on their journey. Obré was in high dudgeon at the way he had been treated by his friend, but after listening to much abuse for his conduct, Richards quietly said to him, "Do you think that I was going to allow you to boast in the club tomorrow how you got off while Richards was robbed!''

For many years after the hospital was opened there was no room set apart specially for operations. In 1775 the need for some such room was beginning to be felt, and a committee set up by the governors did not come to any decision until 1786. Then a room over the west gateway was converted into an operating room at a cost of thirty pounds. The room in question was described as "a small room without any chimney" and it was there that Colles and Cusack afterwards performed many of their brilliant operations. In 1796 John Leigh, the treasurer of the hospital, presented "a convenient chair for the use of the operating theatre". This chair of wood, resembling a dentists' chair, is still preserved in the hospital board-room. That small room on the second landing was not only unsuitable for the actual operations, but more space was urgently required to accommodate the students and spectators who came in considerable numbers to see the surgical operations of that distinguished surgical team. Not infrequently the operator was incommoded by the crush of the spectators who desired to get the closest possible view of every detail of the operation. In 1812 the governors bought, at the cost of £1 12s. 4d., an operating table to supplement the convenient chair given in the previous century by John Leigh. This table was until recently in the hospital, and on it were to be seen the attachments for the straps by which the patients were secured. In 1814 the building of a more commodious theatre was considered by the governors, with Cusack superintending its erection, and it appears to have been completed in 1825, costing about five hundred pounds, Colles and his colleagues each contributing twenty-five pounds towards the building fund. The theatre then built continued in use till the present one was substituted for it in 1896. It formed an extension from the hospital over the west gateway, the entrance being from the middle corridor through the old operating room. The wooden seats for the students and spectators were arranged along the western wall, and from them an excellent view of the operation could be obtained. In its arrangement, like other operating rooms of the time, it resembled more a lecture theatre than a modern operating theatre, and there were, of course, few facilities for surgical cleanliness as it is at present understood. In spite of its drawback, many generations of students watched from its benches some of the most brilliant surgeons in Ireland operate, both before and after the introduction of surgical anaesthesia, and the birth of antiseptic surgery. The care of the theatre was put under the charge of the nurse of No. 7 ward, who was to "be responsible for its general cleanliness, and who shall see that nurses clear away the sawdust, etc. after each operation from their respective wards". The plan, however, did not work well, and a year later Nurse Clinton, who had charge of the operating theatre, was dismissed and five shillings a quarter was paid to one of the assistants, in addition to the usual wages "for keeping the operation theatre in proper order, the matron to keep the key."

Nurse Clinton and her kind, who had care of the patients, occupied a very different position from those of the present day. One nurse was appointed to each ward. Her duties were to collect the medicines from the resident surgeon and administer them as directed, to keep the ward clean and tidy, to wash the bandages and the bed-linen, to collect the provisions from the steward and take them to the cook, to feed the patients and to clean and tidy the rooms for the apprentices and pupils. For this she received £12 yearly, free lodgings, with some furniture, but had to pay for her own food. The nurses often signed the receipt for their wages with their mark, being evidently unable to write even their names. A nurse and her assistant were responsible for a ward of about twenty patients. She lived in the nurse's room off the ward, and there she might house a friend or relative, who acted as her assistant. Occasionally a husband was included in the menage, but children were not allowed. Accommodation in the room was inadequate and the establishment of different families in various parts of the hospital was bound to cause trouble. Thefts of patients' food and belongings was commonplace. The governors, medical staff, matron and steward all in turn appear to have hired and dismissed the nurses. As late as 1855 the first rule was "that the nurses and resident servants be free from the burden of families, and be able to read and write". By then Florence Nightingale and her band of nurses had arrived in the Crimea, and decades more had to pass before these "Nightingales" were to grace the wards and corridors of the hospital, and also the pages of J. Johnston Abraham's *The Night Nurse*.

In 1910, Mrs. William Colles presented a pulpit and reading desk to the new chapel in memory of Abraham and William Colles, father and son, who were connected with the hospital for one hundred years.

CHAPTER 6

Colles and his Contemporaries

"Great men grow as we recede from them"

For Ireland the eighteenth century was to end ingloriously in rebellion and in the Act of Union, and Dublin was now to undergo rapid social and economic changes not unlike those that befell Scotland's capital almost a century before. To quote McDowell—"Dublin's great century ended abruptly on the 1st January, 1801, when the Act of Union came into force. The city ceased to be a parliamentary capital and its social glories were thereby sadly diminished. In 1800, about ninety temporal and spiritual peers resided in Dublin. By 1830 the number had shrunk to eighteen and by 1900 to five, and the Dublin season, when shorn of its dignity and excitement of a parliamentary session, lost much of its attraction. Moreover, the change in Dublin's status must have affected the morale alike of the sensitive and ambitious. Artistic appreciation provides a doubtful basis on which to assess public opinion, but it is difficult to abstain from commenting on the difference between Malton's views, published 1792–1797, and Brocas' views of 1820. Malton portrays a city which is consciously a capital. Over his proud array of public buildings there hangs an air of melancholy grandeur. Brocas, a brisk but insensitive draughtsman, pictures a bustling, cheerful, slightly vulgar provincial city, and it is perhaps of more significance that the two most striking literary figures of the early nineteenth-century Dublin, Maturin and Mangan, are fascinated by ruin and decay."

At the beginning of the new century Ireland's population was about four million, of whom two hundred thousand resided in the capital. With the exodus of the aristocracy there was a corresponding increase in the social status of the professional classes. The doctors were now found residing in the best streets and squares, withdrawing from the second-class streets, such as Stephen Street, Bishop Street, Grafton Street, Jervis Street, Suffolk Street and William Street, in which they lived for many decades before the Union. Gamble tells us, "Dublin's physicians do not forget that they are men and Irishmen—they converse, laugh and drink, and have thrown aside the grave airs and formal manners with the large wigs and gold-headed canes of their predecessors: they have a candour and openness of address, an ease and dignity of deportment, far superior to their London brethren—the truth is, a physician here is almost at the pinnacle of greatness: there are few resident nobility or gentry since the Union, and the professors of law and medicine may be said to form the aristocracy of the place." But most authorities agree with William Stokes that in the first quarter of the nineteenth century the mind of Ireland was sunk in apathy and dejection and there was a marked decline in intellectual vitality. It was in the later period, 1830–1850, that a singular development of intellect and energy took place in every department of mental culture, under the names of George Petrie, Frederick Burton, Samuel Ferguson, Thomas Davis, Clarence Mangan, Rowan Hamilton and James McCullogh.

In April 1813, the Army Medical Board addressed a letter to the Royal College of Surgeons in Ireland, stating that their diploma would be received as a proof of surgical ability in candidates seeking employment in the medical department of the Army, but pointed out that the department always required proof of a medical education as well as a surgical one. The receipt of this letter determined the College to institute forthwith a chair in the practice of Physic, of which the first occupant was the celebrated Dr. John Cheyne.

John Cheyne was born in Leith near Edinburgh in 1777, where his father was a doctor. He entered Edinburgh University in his fifteenth year, and graduated M.D. in June 1795 in his eighteenth year. Having already passed an examination at Surgeons' Hall, he immediately joined the Army as an assistant surgeon, and went with the Horse Artillery to Ireland where he was present at Vinegar Hill in the 1798 Rebellion; although he admits his days were spent "in shooting, playing billiards, and in complete dissipation of time". Returning to Edinburgh, he studied pathology under Charles Bell, and later settled in Dublin in 1809, where he found "the profession respected and its physicians eminent". Smith, Barry, Quinn and Percival were then the leaders, and were mostly of the school of Cullen. They relied chiefly on the accuracy of symptomatology and paid but little attention to morbid anatomy. From November, 1810, to May, 1811, Cheyne received only three guineas in fees. In 1811 he was appointed physician to the Meath Hospital and in the following year his fees amounted to £472. In 1815 he was appointed physician to the House of Industry, where he had charge of upwards of 70 patients with acute diseases, mainly fevers. "Only eight or ten of these demanded careful examination—the rest of the patients required only a glance of the eye, so that the visit was always finished in little more than an hour." In 1816 his income was £1700 a year and rapidly rose to £5000. He was now doing so well in private practice that he resigned his professorship of the Surgeons' School in 1819, and also his appointment at the Meath Hospital. His colleague, Edward Percival, at the House of Industry, who arrived in Dublin with Cheyne and equally penniless, was now averaging £7000 per annum, and shortly afterwards retired in comfort to Bath. Cheyne succeeded Percival as Physician-General in 1820 and was the last holder of that lucrative office, which was abolished on his retirement in 1833. The last ten years of Cheyne's professional life in Dublin were clouded by mental strain or "nervous fever" and he took himself to religion on retirement to England, where he died in 1836. His rather strange book, *Essays on the partial derangement of the mind in supposed connection with religion*, published posthumously in 1843, is interpreted as an apology and atonement for his worldly successes, and also contains his autobiography. Cheyne is remembered for his description (1818) associated with William Stokes, of the respiration now known to us as "Cheyne-Stokes Respiration".

Cheyne, Colles, Percival and Todd introduced in 1817 a new medical journal styled *Dublin Hospital Reports and communications in Medicine and Surgery*. Dublin at that time had no medical journal, as its first journal, the *Dublin Medical and Physical Essays*, published ten years previously, failed after eighteen

months, having issued only six numbers, and the Dublin
medical profession had to publish their papers in the *Edinburgh
Medical and Surgical Journal*—then the leading medical journal
of the age. The latter journal paid this graceful tribute to its
new competitor (1817):

> "We have great satisfaction in introducing this volume
> to the attention of our readers, as one of the most valuable
> which has been published since we began our critical labours.
> Excellent as it is, we trust that it is only the first of a long
> series, and we shall have to bestow still higher commendation
> upon each succeeding volume.
>
> "The title is not, however, accurately descriptive of the
> nature of the work, for although "Dublin Hospital Reports"
> occupy a distinguished part, yet it contains many papers
> which owe their origin to private practice and to observation
> unconnected with Dublin. In point of fact, its plan coincides
> with that of the *Medico-Chirurgical Transactions* of London,
> and in the manner in which it has begun to be carried
> into effect, shows, that if Ireland has not hitherto been
> distinguished for its periodical productions in regard to
> the healing art, its backwardness has not been owing to
> deficiency of observation or talent in the profession, but to
> causes over which they had no control—chiefly, we suspect,
> inactivity on the part of the publishers, and an erroneous
> belief that Ireland could not support a periodical work.
> This volume above is calculated to dissipate that illusion,
> and now that our brethren on the other side of the Channel
> have proved their strength, they will be to blame if they
> allow it again to obscure their merit. But we must hasten
> the truth of our eulogism, which everyone must consider as
> disinterested, since this publication will deprive us, at least,
> of the elaborate papers of many valuable correspondents."

Subsequent volumes of the *Dublin Hospital Reports* appeared
at irregular intervals, in 1818, 1822 and 1827, with Cheyne
and Colles as editors, and the final volume was edited by
Graves in 1830. Colles contributed papers to all five volumes.
When John Cheyne resigned the chair of medicine in the

Surgeons' School in 1819, Whitley Stokes succeeded him. Stokes, described by "Erinensis" as "patriot, scholar and an *Irishman*" and acclaimed by Wolfe Tone "as the very best man he had ever known", had incurred Lord Clare's enmity in 1798 and was for three years passed over for advancement to senior fellowship in Trinity. Later he was to resign this fellowship to become professor of natural history. He was now physician to the Meath Hospital and was succeeded there by his son William—"the great Stokes", who was also to succeed his father in the Regius chair of Physic in Trinity later. Whitley Stokes was in Edinburgh during Colles' sojourn there, but he only attended one clinical session in 1795–96 and did not matriculate or graduate in that University.

The leading surgeon at the Meath Hospital was Philip Crampton who, as a young man, had succeeded William Dease in 1798. Crampton, four times president of his College, Surgeon-General in 1813, baronet in 1839, was probably Colles' nearest rival. In 1804 he established the first of the private medical schools and taught anatomy and surgery at the rear of his house in Dawson Street. An able anatomist and surgeon, flamboyant in character, always moving in high society, he enjoyed much publicity during his long career. A circumstance which occurred in 1810 made him the subject of town talk for a considerable time, and, it is said, had an immediate effect on his practice. A waiter in the Richmond Tavern, which was situated opposite to Crampton's house, was choking from the impaction of a piece of meat in his oesophagus. Crampton was sent for and promptly performed tracheostomy and the man recovered. "Erinensis" naturally had much material for his biographical sketch on Crampton.

"For of his immediate kindred he is the most important himself; and of his ancestors by far the most important that we could hear of were Adam and Eve. From this venerable couple he is descended in a direct line. About six feet in height, slightly formed, elegantly proportioned, and elastic as corkwood. If, instead of the gothic fabric by which his graceful figure was distorted, he had been habitated in flowing robes of Lincoln green, he must doubtless have passed for the model of James FitzJames. A blue coat, with scarcely anything deserving the name of skirts, a pair of doeskin breeches that did every justice to the ingenious maker, top boots, spurs of imposing longitude, and a whip called a 'blazer' in his country, completed the costume of this dandy Nimrod. Lord Whitworth, at this period Viceroy of Ireland, happened to be seized by one of those bowel complaints which nature very often inflicts upon gluttons, as a chastisement for the violation of her laws. Mr. Crampton was, of course, called in. All remedies had been tried—they all failed and the vital spark was hastening fast to extinction; when, Lo! the invincible hero of our story puts off his 'woollens', jumps into bed, and grapples with death face to face in the body of the moribund Lord. The calories radiating from Crampton's warm heart reanimated his expiring patient and just infused into his feeble arm sufficient strength to sign a draft of £500 on the Bank of Ireland, to be paid to Mr. Crampton as a trifling remuneration for his devoted attention. Surely this ingenious and magnanimous mode of treatment deserved no less a reward. In the whole routine of medical practice we have never heard of anything to equal this. Heroes, to be sure, have died for their country, lovers for their lasses, and friendship has had its force demonstrated by the attachment of Damon and Phintias, but, avaunt, Romance! where shall we find in thy world of wonders, love so disinterested and sincere, so profound as this attempt to restore the dying by a combination of those powers applied in the novel but elegant formula of an animal fomentation? The sublimity of this act could not be lost upon an admiring world, for who is there amongst us who would not have that man for a medical attendant, who would thus lay aside the dignity of his profession with his garments, to sooth the pangs of disease and 'to return sigh for sigh?'. In addition to the £500, the noble Lord, on his recovery, presented Mr. Crampton with a general's uniform, in which he shortly appeared in the Castle of Dublin. Lord Norbury was one of the party, but so completely had the new apparel transformed his old acquaintance that he asked a gentleman standing by him, who was that who wore the general's uniform?

The gentleman observed it was the Surgeon-General. 'Oh, yes,' replied the witty Lord jocusely, who was never at a loss for a pun or a halter, 'I suppose that is the General of the Lancers!' . . .

". . . We happened to be present, some time back, at one of those scenes of scientific butchery at the Meath Hospital. The patient was a female. The complaint, if we recollect rightly, open scrofula of the knee-joint. A great concourse assembled to witness the operation. It was quite a gala day with the dissectors—a festival seemingly held in honour of the virtues of *Steel*. It was the first time, we believe, that the removal of the knee-joint was attempted here; we earnestly hope it will be the last. The operator (Crampton), of course, accomplished his purpose with his usual dexterity. But could he have beheld, as we did, the contorted countenances of his spectators, the knife would have fallen from his hand, never to be resumed where it was not more imperiously indicated. To be present was indeed to be in torture. One man vented his feelings in a *wink*, the second in a *hem*, a third overcame his sympathies in a forced fit of laughter, a fourth put his fingers in his ears to shut out the wretch's screams. All, to be sure, admired, yet all disapproved, and before the performance was entirely finished, Colles cried out in rather an audible tone, 'By Jayshus',* drew the door after him and vanished."

Crampton was the first surgeon in Dublin to perform lithrotrity in 1834 and insisted that it should be the procedure of choice. Dr. Civiale is usually regarded as the inventor of the lithrotrite and it was his instrument with its many modifications, especially by L'Estrange of Dublin, that was now in use. There is, however, evidence that the procedure of crushing the bladder stone was carried out as early as 15 A.D. by Ammonius of Alexandria, and Crampton resurrected an interesting account of the procedure being employed in Dublin in 1539

* "The plainer Dubliners amaze us
   By their frequent use of Jaysus
   Which makes us entertain the notion
   It is not always from devotion."
                              Oliver St. John Gogarty, 1937.

with Sir Herbert Sidney, the Lord President, as the patient. Colles and the other Dublin surgeons, however, still preferred the classical operation of lateral lithotomy as introduced and practised with success by Frère Jacques and Cheselden, though now modified by the use of the lithotome in which the knife was introduced via a grooved staff. One such lithotome was invented in 1750 by George Daunt, surgeon to Mercer's Hospital, Dublin, and for which he received the thanks and congratulations of the Royal Academy of Surgery of Paris in 1775. Daunt, a bold operator, is remembered by Gilborne:

> "Undaunted Daunt in rank is foremost
> His operations nice our Annals fill
> His well-contrived discoveries of note
> Improve the Art and Mankind's good promote."

William Dease improved on Daunt's lithotome and became expert in its use. Colles said in a kind reference to him, "Old Mr. Dease was in the habit of constantly performing the motions his hands would take in this manoeuvre; even at the dinner table, while speaking to someone, he might often be detected moving his knife and fork as if pushing the scalpel and staff on together without thinking of what he was doing." Dease was often accused by his imitators of keeping a stone conveniently in his pocket in case his diagnosis was wrong and also of not disclosing his method of operating. Crampton protested vehemently against these accusations and upheld the honour of his old chief and Father of Irish Surgery.

Robert Moore Peile improved on the instrument still further and at one time "Peile's lithotome and staff" were to be found in every surgery. Professor Robert Smith stated that, out of the forty operations for stone which he knew to have been performed by Peile, only one had a fatal result. Peile, elected a member at the first meeting of the College, lived to be about ninety-six and outlived by several years all the original members of the College. He was for over fifty years surgeon to the House of Industry and was also consultant surgeon to Dr. Steevens' Hospital, where he acted as assistant to Colles when the latter was tying the subclavian artery. His disposition was singularly gentle and he was never known to betray anger or impatience. Shortly before his death, his friend and former pupil, Dr. Bigger, was trying to induce him to swallow some wine jelly. Peile said, in his usual gentle manner, "Now, my dear friend, will you be good enough to permit me to die." He smiled upon those around his bedside and shortly afterwards expired. "Metropolis" thought kindly of Peile when he penned the following lines:

> "Ingratiating manners, feeling, mind,
> His hand as steady as his heart is kind,
> Thro' pathless darkness, dubious and untried,
> Like him the desp'rate Gorget who can guide?
> Or steal, with delicacy's touch, away
> The lens, whose cloud obscures the visual ray."

The name of Robert James Graves (of the disease) is familiar to all medical men. He was the most dynamic medical personality ever produced by his country, and he revolutionised the teaching of medicine in these islands. The descendant of one of Cromwell's colonels who had, in the polite parlance of Victorian biographers, "acquired considerable property in the county of Limerick", Graves was born in Dublin in 1797, where his father was senior fellow and Regius professor of Divinity at Trinity. Young Graves had a phenomenal career in its medical school, having taken every possible prize in his course on the way to his degree in 1818. He then spent three years in foreign travel, visiting medical centres in London, Edinburgh, France, Germany and Italy. His faculty for languages was such that in Austria he was taken for a German spy and had to submit to ten days' imprisonment before his correct identification procured his release. Crossing the Alps on foot en route for Italy, he shared the company of Turner the artist. They travelled together for weeks, stopping at the same inns, eating, conversing and sketching together, neither asking the other's name until it was time to part company. Once, sailing from Genoa to Sicily, his ship ran into a storm, its sails torn to ribbons, its pumps choked, and its crew about to cast off in a rowing boat prepared to leave the passengers to their fate; Graves, though

abominably seasick, seized an axe and stove in the sides of the
rowing boat, declaring it was "a pity to break up such good
company". Then, taking command of the stricken crew, he
had the suckers of the pumps removed, and cutting from his
own boots the leather necessary, had its valves renewed. The
crew returned to their duties, the leak was stopped and the
vessel saved. Back in Dublin he was appointed physician to
the Meath Hospital in 1821, and to Whitley Stokes, his senior
colleague there, the coming of this remarkably outspoken man
must have been comparable to the sudden blast of a whirlwind
down its hitherto peaceful corridors. Graves' opening lecture at
the Meath Hospital shook the complacency of the Dublin pundits
severely. He contrasted the manners of Irish physicians with
those of the French, very much to the disadvantage of the former.
He spoke of the "laudable curiosity on the part of the students,
suppressed by a forbidding demeanour or an incourteous
answer from his teacher", and again of French physicians,
"We do not find them indulging in coarse, harsh, and even
vulgar expressions to their hospital patients; we do not find them
with two vocabularies—one for the rich and another for the
poor." Many lives, he boldly declared, were lost each year
owing to bad treatment by doctors whose teachers had never
taught them to practise: students "walking the hospitals" in
Dublin made their appearance there as critics rather than as
learners, coming to hospitals seeking entertainment, rather
than instruction. Many were annually dubbed doctors who
had scarcely ever been called upon to write a prescription—
practitioners these who had never practised, whose errors were
to grow with the years for the want of properly directed clinical
instruction in their youth. The hospital lectures given before
his time, both in Edinburgh and Dublin, consisted of Olympian
dissertations, delivered in indifferent Latin by a lecturer to a
class who, notebook in hand, took down and memorised his
every word. That aristocratic gulf between teacher and pupil
was broken down by Graves. The practice of medicine, he
declared, could not be learned by hearsay: this was "book
medicine" at its very worst. Taking his class to the bedside, he
allotted to each student a patient, every detail of whose course
was to be studied and recorded from beginning to end of his

stay in hospital. Graves' *student practitioner* was thus charged with the personal responsibility of investigating his cases for himself and by himself, under the personal guidance of the teacher. The clinical methods taught in all medical schools today we owe to Graves. Of his numerous publications, perhaps his *Clinical lectures on the practice of Medicine* (1848) is the most famous; it was received with general acclamation in the most widely-spread medical circles, and earned the plaudits of the great Trousseau. Graves was elected King's professor of the Institutes of Medicine in 1827 in the School of Physic and gave lectures in Sir Patrick Dun's Hospital. He was the founder and first president of the Pathological Society of Dublin and was succeeded in that office by Colles. Graves and Colles were close friends and one is not surprised to read that Colles' youngest son bore the Christian name of Graves. Robert Graves retired and died at the early age of fifty-six, and across the century comes back his voice, speaking in his retirement: "A short and transitory existence has been allotted to out bodies; individuals die, generations pass away, but the common intellect of mankind fears not the same fate, nor shares the same brief mortality."

William Stokes, like Graves, requires no introduction to the medical reader. William was the son of Whitley Stokes and was born in Dublin in 1804. His early education was conducted at home under the eye of his father, his tutor being John Walker, an ex-fellow of Trinity, who founded the Walkerite sect already referred to. His father was a strong-minded adherent to the Dissenting Communion, and a letter addressed to his wife reads: "I think they (his sons) should be well acquainted with the Latin language, botany and chemistry, and acquainted also with ancient and modern history will make them be the judges of value of the Holy Scriptures and more convinced of their truth. I would not have them sent to school or college, and would rather have them very ignorant than that they should purchase knowledge at the price of corruption of their morals." Further advantages were that William met brilliant intellects in his father's home, "especially when outside was ill-ordered, indolent society, dejected, discontented, inert, and more mournful than all, indifferent to aught but selfish and petty intrigue". William was a constant companion to his father and assisted him in his natural history lectures in Trinity. After a short preliminary course of study at the Surgeons' School under Colles and in the chemistry department of professor Barker in Trinity, he left for Glasgow to complete his chemistry studies in professor Thomson's department. Later, Stokes went to Edinburgh to complete his medical education under professor Alison and graduated there in 1825. But before graduation he had already published a small volume on the use of the stethoscope. Appointed physician to the Meath Hospital, to succeed his father, he began a life-long friendship with Graves as his colleague. Together they developed that clinical teaching of medicine that made the Meath Hospital famous in the annals of medicine. His two books, *Diseases of the Lungs and Windpipe*, 1837, and *Diseases of the Heart and Aorta*, 1854, are classics in the literature of our profession. In the latter work there is an abridged account of the postmortem findings on the body of Abraham Colles, which is prefaced as follows: "I will give the case of my venerated friend and teacher, the late Mr. Colles, who so long filled the chair of surgery in the Royal College of Surgeons in Ireland. The case of this remarkable man and eminent surgeon was published by me in 1846, but I believe that in inserting it in this work, though in an abridged form, I shall be acting in accordance with the expressed desire of Mr. Colles, that the history of his case should be, as far as possible, made available for the advancement of medicine." It was in this volume also that we read the description of that form of respiration associated with his name and that of another great Irish physician, John Cheyne. "A form of respiratory distress, peculiar to this affection (fatty degeneration of the heart) consisting of a period of apparently perfect apnoea, succeeded by feeble and short inspirations, which gradually increase in strength and depth, until the respiratory act is carried to the highest pitch of which it seems capable. When the respirations pursuing a descending scale, regularly diminish until the commencement of another apnoeal period. During the height of the paroxysm the vesicular murmur becomes intensely puerile." William Stokes is also remembered in association with Robert Adams for the description (1846) of the permanently

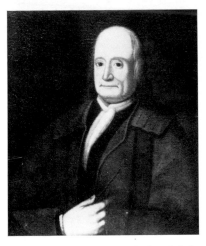

Fig. 1 William Colles of Kilcollen (1648-1719) Eminent surgeon of Kilkenny. Great grandfather of Abraham Colles

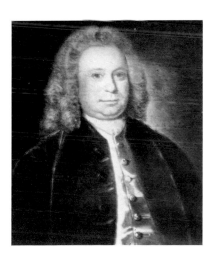

Fig. 2 William Colles of Abbeyvale (1702-1770). Distinguished citizen and mayor of Kilkenny. He developed the family marble business. Grandfather of Abraham Colles

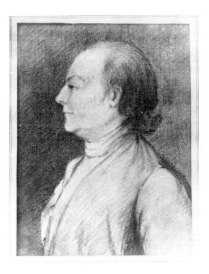

Fig. 3 William Colles of Millmount (1745-1779). Built Millmount in 1770. Married Mary Anne Bates in 1771, and carried on the family marble business. Father of Abraham Colles

Figs. 1, 2 & 3. Reproduced by courtesy of Sir Dudley Colles.

[Facing page 130

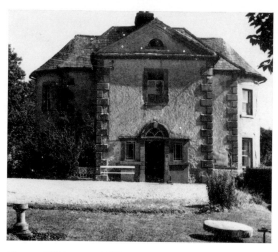

Fig. 4 Millmount, Kilkenny. Built by William Colles
(1745-1779) in 1770. Abraham Colles was born here in
1773. Photograph by courtesy of "the Kilkenny people"

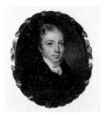

Fig. 5 Abraham
Colles as a young
man from a minia-
ture in possession of
Ronald M. Colles

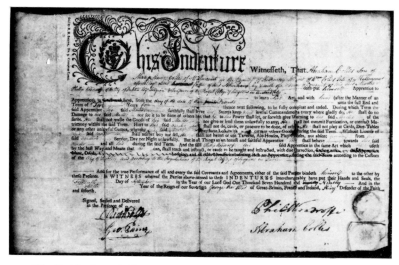

Fig. 6 Abraham Colles Indenture Certificate 15th September 1790

Fig. 6. Reproduced by courtesy of R.C.S.I.

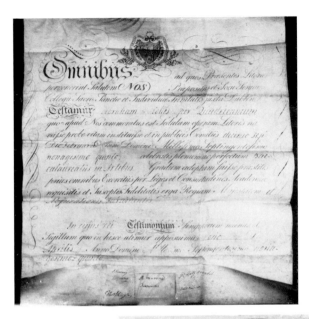

Fig. 7 Abraham Colles B.A. Diploma 9th April 1795 Trinity College, University of Dublin

Fig. 8 "Letters Testimonial" or Licence Royal College of Surgeons in Ireland 24th September 1795

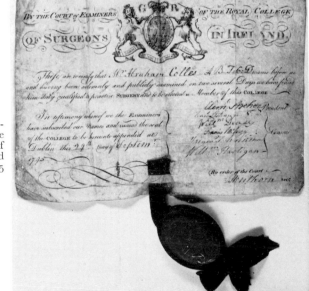

Fig. 7. Reproduced by courtesy of Mrs. George Lucas.

Fig. 8. Reproduced by courtesy of R.C.S.I.

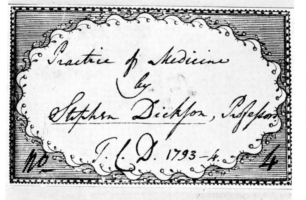

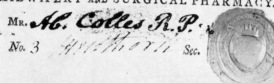

Fig. 9 Abraham Colles Class Admission Tickets 1. Royal College of Surgeons in Ireland 2. Trinity College, Dublin 3. University of Edinburgh

Fig. 9. Reproduced by courtesy of Mrs. George Lucas.

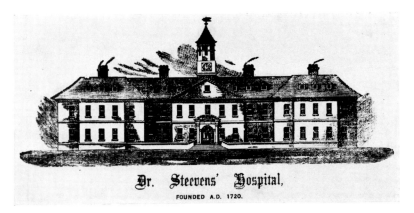

(a)

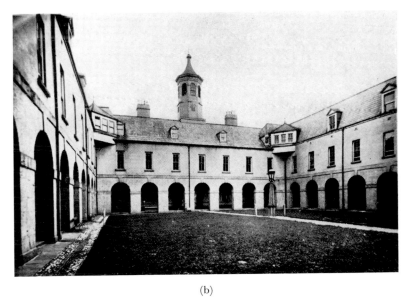

(b)

Fig. 10 (a) Dr. Steevens' Hospital, Dublin founded in 1720. (b) The quadrangle, looking east

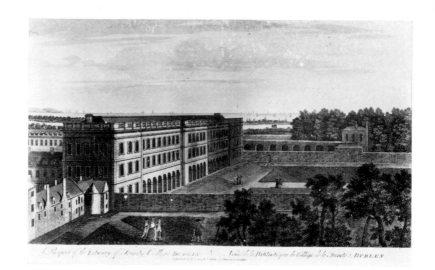

Fig. 11. An eighteenth-century print of Trinity College, Dublin. Library, and its first Medical School, right foreground, opened in 1711

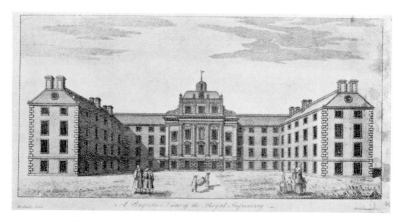

Fig. 12 Royal Infirmary, Edinburgh, founded in 1738

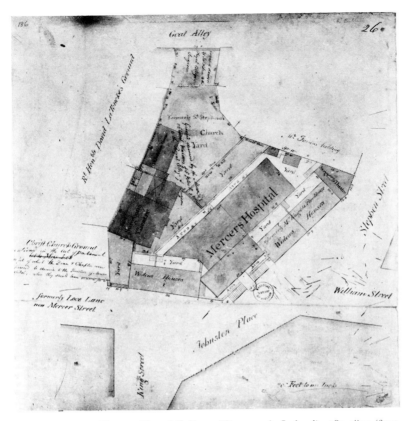

Fig. 13 Surgeons Theatre (Royal College of Surgeons in Ireland) 1789-1810 (from the Longfield Collection National Library of Ireland)

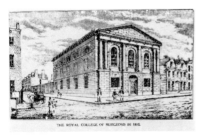

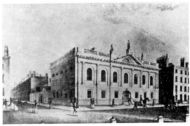

Fig. 14 Royal College of Surgeons in Ireland in 1810.

Fig. 15 Engraving of The Royal College of Surgeons in Ireland on its completion in 1827

Figs. 14 & 15. Reproduced by courtesy of R.C.S.I.

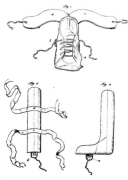

Fig. 16 The Colles' apparatus for the treatment of Varus or Club Feet in infants

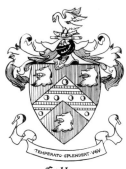

Colles.

Fig. 17 The Colles family crest and coat of arms

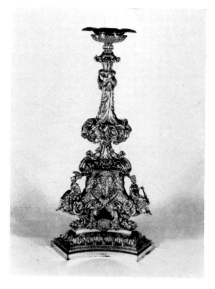

Fig. 18 A table centre-piece in silver, 30 inches high, weighing 27 pounds. Inscribed—"Presented by the Royal College of Surgeons in Ireland to Abraham Colles, Esq., in gratitude for services rendered while Professor to the School of Surgery in this country, and in testimony of esteem for professional worth and integrity. Dublin 1838"

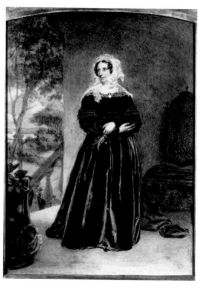

Fig. 19 Sophia Cope (1782-1858). Daughter of Rev. Jonathan Cope of Ahascragh, Co. Galway. Granddaughter of Henry Cope M.D. of Dublin (1684-1743). State Physician 1733. Descendant of Sir Anthony Cope, Vice-Chamberlain to Catherine Parr (1512-1548). Married Abraham Colles on 25th April 1807

Fig. 18. Reproduced by courtesy of Ronald M. Colles.

Fig. 19. Reproduced by courtesy of Sir Dudley Colles.

slow pulse—"the Stokes-Adams syndrome". The subsequent career of William Stokes in the Regius chair of Physic in Trinity, which he occupied for thirty-eight years, during which time he was described by Sir George Paget, Regius professor of Physic at Cambridge, as "the greatest physician of that time in Europe", are outwith the scope of this memoir. But there is a passage in a letter that William Stokes wrote to his wife in 1829 which, unfortunately, still holds a message for his fellow countrymen. "Oh, that we could all unite in striving for civil and religious liberty, that this fair land for which God has done so much and man so little, might put forth its smothered energies which now burst forth only to ruin and destroy."

When Richard Dease, Colles' co-professor in the chairs of anatomy and surgery, died in 1819 as a result of a wound received in the dissecting room, Charles Hawkes Todd was appointed to fill the vacancy and shared both chairs with Colles until 1826. Todd was surgeon to the House of Industry, and was probably the first to suggest the radical cure of aneurysm by compression. He was much and deservedly esteemed for the accuracy of his anatomical knowledge and for the clear and concise manner in which he communicated that knowledge to his pupils. So minute indeed were his demonstrations that it is said that the vertebral and other ligaments expanded to a degree beyond what nature had intended! "Erinensis" presents him "full, fat and forty" for biographical consideration.

"His robust frame, rustic features, and ruddy complexion, along with other corresponding charms, would do equal honour to the hale member of a farming society, or to the beef and claret amateur of a city corporation. His sleek well fed person, is a most appropriate illustration of the *ventri obedienta* of Sallust. The table behind which he stands is no longer a *tabula rasa*, with nothing to relieve the eye from the uniformity of the scene, save the refreshing verdure of some green baize. It is now daily strewn with those varieties which, forsooth, excel, in point of execution, even continental ingenuity; all of which Mr. Todd arranged in 'gay theatric pride', with so much precision as an experienced butler collocates the intricate furniture of an epicure's dinner service. To this array of morbid preserves, a watch is added as if the speaker was about to run a race with time, or to measure his discourse by the revolution of the minute hand. Everything being at length adjusted to the professor's satisfaction, he patiently waits until the *Exquisites* have drawn up their spear-pointed shirt necks, frizzed up their curls, settled their umbrellas, and until the last echoes of the brazen boot-heels and clanking of chains have died away among the benches. The moment of inspiration commences, the speaker immunges his nose with all his might, a doleful voice, scarcely audible, something like the melancholy moan of the midnight breeze, which so few have heard, informs you that the person whom you might have supposed destitute of the organs of speech, possesses in some respects the faculty of speaking. As yet all is little more than dumb show and pantomimic solemnity. By degrees a few inspirations bring the vocal organs into a more perfect state of modulation, while each word, separated from its fellow by a considerable hiatus, is followed up *pari passu*, with a delectable accompaniment, reverberated through the mazy labyrinths of the nose. The invariable monotony of the Gregorian note can only rival the sing-song solemnity of this surgical ditty. In vain you expect the importance of the subject, the presence of an audience, and the situation of the speaker would call forth some animated exertion. But his narrative is never enlivened by any of those practical anecdotes and *double entendres* with which Mr. Colles occasionally sets his hearers in roars of laughter. He does not possess the same colloquial fluency or tact of discrimination which are the principal attractions in the lectures of the latter gentleman."

Todd lived at No. 3 Kildare Street, where the Kildare Street Club now stands. He died in 1826 at the early age of forty-four. All his fifteen children reached adult age and all save one married. One of his sons, Robert Bentley Todd, became professor of physiology and morbid anatomy at King's College Hospital Medical School, London. He was also physician to that hospital and his statue now adorns its forecourt. In addition to numerous publications, he projected the famous *Cyclopaedia of Anatomy and Physiology* (1835–1859).

When Colles resigned the post of resident surgeon at Dr. Steevens' Hospital in February 1813 and was appointed assistant surgeon, James William Cusack was elected resident surgeon in his place. Up to that time and in the eighty years of its history, there were only four resident surgeons, Lewis (dismissed), Butler, Woodroffe and Colles, and it is of interest that Woodroffe, Colles and Cusack were presidents of their College during their period of office as resident surgeons to the hospital. Cusack had been apprenticed to Obré and was a student of the Surgeons' School and at Dr. Steevens' Hospital. He was also a matriculated student at Trinity and had a distinguished career in the arts and medical courses. Cusack had a large practice, especially after Colles' death, when he became the leading surgeon in Ireland. He also had an unusually great number of apprentices, due mainly to his connection with the Park Street medical School of which he was a founder. When his apprentices attained the number of fifty-two, his pupils styled him "Colonel of the 52nd". He was a most hospitable man, particularly in the case of his former apprentices and his home at No. 9 Kildare Street, formerly owned by Todd, was always an open one. At one time eleven of the surgeons of county infirmaries were his past apprentices. It was while Cusack was resident surgeon that Charles Lever, the novelist, was a student of the hospital, and there he played many of those practical jokes which he has described in *Charles O'Malley*; where Lever makes Frank Webber personate Doctor Mooney, one of the tutors in Trinity, and this is founded on one of the incidents that took place in the hospital. It was the custom of Cusack, like Prodicus, the Cean at Athens, to make his pupils attend him in his bedroom each morning before he got up, in order to question them about their work and to give them such clinical instruction as he thought fit. This was Cusack's happy interpretation of that "bedside" teaching, later to be successfully inaugurated by Graves and Stokes at the Meath Hospital. The ideas of clinical instruction have altered somewhat since that time and it is difficult now to imagine a class of students attending to receive instruction while their master lies in bed. Cusack, however,

seems to have had no difficulty in enforcing the rule. One night
Cusack was called unexpectedly from the hospital and in the
morning Lever learned that he had not returned. Having
instructed the hospital porter to say nothing of the resident
surgeon's absence, Lever got into Cusack's bed and, putting on
his red silk nightcap, received the class in the manner of the
original owner. The joke was carried on for some time before
Lever disclosed his identity, and he was so popular with his
fellow students that he escaped any serious consequence from it.
Although fond of practical jokes, Lever was a favourite with his
teachers, and Cusack, in particular, seems to have allowed him
great freedom. Cusack disliked tobacco smoke and strict
orders were made that no one was to smoke within the
precincts of the hospital. One afternoon Cusack, on going to
No. 1 ward, saw a man in bed at the far end of the ward, smoking a pipe. The patient, seeing Cusack, at once lay down and
pretended to be asleep. Cusack went up to him and accused him
of smoking, which the patient promptly denied. The denial was
not accepted and a nurse was called and she was directed to
search the bed for the offending pipe. The search was fruitless
and Cusack had to leave, discomfited and unconvinced. So
satisfied was he that he had seen the pipe that he returned and
said to the man that if he told him what he had done with the
pipe, the matter would be dropped. The patient told him to try
his own pocket and there the pipe was found, the man having
slipped it in while Cusack was calling for the nurse. Cusack
enjoyed the joke as much as anyone. Cusack worried much
about his operations and lay awake at night before his operation
day, pondering over details of his cases. He published very
little, but his ability as a surgeon cannot be questioned. In the
Dublin Hospital Reports, 1817, he described a case of a woman
aged thirty-six, suffering from sarcoma of the lower jaw. Having tied the carotid artery, Cusack proceeded to the excision
of half the lower jaw. This patient underwent the ordeal, of
nearly an hour's duration, sitting in that "convenient chair"
and, at the close of the operation "courteously declining assistance, walked to her bed". These patients showed an amazing
fortitude. Ten years later Cusack published in the same
journal a series of seven such resections of the lower jaw, with

one fatality. Years after Colles' death, Cusack was appointed in 1852 to a second chair—the University professorship of surgery in Trinity—which title was altered to the Regius professorship of surgery (1868) during the tenure of its next occupant, Robert Adams (of the "Stokes-Adams syndrome"). Cusack was president of his College on three occasions, in 1827, 1847 and 1858.

Samuel Wilmot was exactly contemporary with Colles. They entered Trinity together as students in the same year (1790), but Wilmot's father, who had an aversion to surgery, insisted that his son, who desired to study the healing art, confine himself to medicine. On his father's death, however, Wilmot entered the Surgeons' School under Hartigan and received his licence from that College, and later his medical degrees from Trinity. He became assistant surgeon to Jervis Street Hospital, and was deputy to Hartigan in Trinity during the latter's illness. He and his friends assumed that he would succeed Hartigan, although Trinity had made it clear to him that his appointment as deputy was not to establish his right of succession. Macartney was appointed to Hartigan's chair. In 1814 Wilmot succeeded Obré as assistant surgeon to Dr. Steevens' Hospital. It was this team of Colles, Wilmot and Cusack that gave the hospital the leading place in Irish surgery, as Graves and Stokes did for medicine at the Meath Hospital. Wilmot was, for a short while, professor of anatomy in the Surgeons' School after Todd's death. He resigned the Anatomy chair but continued as co-professor of surgery with Colles for a further nine years, when they both resigned that chair in 1836. Wilmot apparently was a very able teacher, and one of the founders of the celebrated Park Street medical School. When Colles and Wilmot resigned the anatomy chair in the Surgeons' School in 1827, they were succeeded by Robert Harrison and Arthur Jacob. Harrison, an Englishman, was apprenticed to Colles, later becoming his demonstrator in the Surgeons' School. He was also his personal and family friend, and married his wife's sister. During his professorship at the Surgeons' School, Harrison published the *Dublin Dissector*, which went to many editions and was for long a favourite manual in the American anatomy schools. Harrison later succeeded Macartney in the Trinity chair of anatomy and chirurgery.

Arthur Jacob was in those days a fiery figure in Irish surgery and medical politics, and had much in common with Thomas Wakley of *The Lancet*. Born in Maryborough in 1790 and apprenticed there to his father, who was surgeon to Queen's County Infirmary; he then entered the Surgeons' School, and became a pupil of Colles at Dr. Steevens' Hospital. He was later to graduate M.D. of Edinburgh University in 1814. After attending the clinics of Lawrence, Brodie and Cooper in London, he returned to Dublin as demonstrator in anatomy with Macartney at Trinity, succeeding Colles in the anatomy chair in the Surgeons' School in 1827. "Erinensis" describes his entry to the lecture hall thus:

"A gentleman of *duodecimo* stature, so neatly habitated, that the affectation of the *simplex munditiis* could not disguise the assumed indifference to toiletic arrangements and exterior appearance, stepped in by a side door and relieved us from suspense. He was harnessed in a pair of spectacles, so admirably fitted to the prominences and depressions of the orbitary processes, that one might have mistaken the whole optical apparatus as the natural production of the parts, or an expansion of the cornea spread out upon a delicate frame of silver wire. Over the springs of this beautiful piece of mechanism, that held the temples fast in "close embrace", hung two luxuriant ringlets of auburn hair, like the tendrils of a vine and writhing into beautiful contortions from the recent application of the actual cautery. Had 'Crispissa' herself o'erlooked each hair, the tresses which we beheld could not have been more tastefully disposed. He advanced up to the table with a buoyant swing, and with such a smirk of self-complacency upon his countenance, just verging on the laughing point, that we would have been pardoned at the moment, if we had taken him for a jolly disciple of Democritus instead of a grave son of Aesculapius. A momentary pause of amazement ensued, but the audience, as if sympathising with his feelings, gave vent to theirs in a loud burst of approbation. *Ingeminant plausu Tyrii, Troesque sequuntur*,* which hemistich we quote in obedience to Mr. Colles's mandate,

* The Carthaginians roared approval and the Trojans followed suit.

that all surgeons should read the classics and, to balance the account, we translate it to show our skill in versification.

"Clap hands, clap hands, old Mother Steevens cries
And straight her sons with discord rend the skies;
While Richmond's corps of dandies and of asses
In depth of sound all rivalry surpasses."

In addition to the Surgeons' anatomy chair, Jacob, together with Cusack, Wilmot, Graves and others, founded the Park Street medical School in 1824. The buildings of this school, at Cusack's suggestion, were erected in the style of a Methodist Meeting House because, as he thought, the school would not last long and the buildings might be more easily disposed of for religious purposes. About 1824 Park Street was the abode of persons leading unvirtuous lives; and when in later years it was purified from its moral filth, its name was changed to Lincoln Place, which it still remains. The school was closed in 1849 when its principal proprietor, Hugh Carlisle, was appointed professor of anatomy in the newly established Queen's College, Belfast. Jacob was also one of the Surgeons' School professors who founded the Royal City of Dublin Hospital in 1832. In conjunction with Henry Maunsell Jacob established in 1838 the *Dublin Medical Press*, and as its editor he was much given to drastic polemical articles, which frequently greatly irritated those against whom they were directed. Jacob was the first to describe the bacillary layer or layer of rods and cones of the retina, which was named not by its discoverer, "Jacob's membrane". He was also the first to describe rodent ulcer, which in Dublin is still referred to as "Jacob's ulcer". Finally, he invented a curved needle for cataract operations, which bears his name. Arthur Jacob was president of his College in 1837 and 1864.

The rapid expansion of medical education from the mid-eighteenth century onwards gave rise to numerous private medical schools in all the great cities. All that was required was a dissecting room, with the appropriate arrangements with the "ressurectionists", a lecture hall, a small chemical laboratory, perhaps a museum and above all an attractive lecturer.

Many of the schools were so efficient that they attracted students away from the official schools of the universities and Surgeons' colleges. The certificates of these schools were recognised by the Service authorities and often by the official schools, and general practice was, of course, free for all. Many of these schools had a brief existence, many amalgamated, some were later absorbed into the official schools but most were to disappear with the passage of the Medical Registration Act of 1858. Dublin had many such private medical schools in the early nineteenth century, but Colles was never attracted away from the Surgeons' School, although many of his colleagues and contemporaries were.

One such private medical school was opened in 1809 by John Timothy Kirby and Alexander Read at the rear of a house in Stephen Street, close to Mercer's Hospital. Part of the house was occupied by a laundress, whose sign-board bore the words "Mangling done here" and the wags of the day said that the sign-board did duty for Kirby and Read as well as for the laundress. The school, which was named the "Theatre of Anatomy", was transferred to No. 28 Peter Street in the following year, where it was styled the "Theatre of Anatomy and School of Surgery" and attracted numerous students. Read retired from the partnership in 1812 and Kirby became sole proprietor of the school. When the Army medical authorities required candidates for surgeoncies to produce evidence of hospital attendance, Kirby set up a small hospital within his school, containing some twelve beds, which he dedicated to St. Peter and St. Bridget. The fees of the pupils were devoted to the expenses of the hospital. The Peter Street school and its hospital enabled Kirby to give complete sets of medical certificates, which met the requirements of the Navy and Army medical departments, and the London and Edinburgh Colleges of Surgeons, but the Dublin College did not recognise them as they insisted on a minimum of twenty beds. Kirby's certificates were well known in London, apparently were freely forged, and, selling at a high price, allowed at least twenty men to enter the Services by these fraudulent means. Kirby left behind an interesting autobiography, which fortunately was retrieved by Cameron. In it he described his boarding-school days in

Waterford under a drunken curate as headmaster. After leaving school he wanted to join the Army and received a commission during the 1798 Rebellion. He immediately changed his mind and entered the Surgeons' School under Halahan, and at the same time entered Trinity with the Reverend John Walker as his tutor. On Walker's resignation to form his own Calvinistic sect, Kirby was transferred to Mr. Davenport, who died a lunatic. After qualification, Kirby was appointed demonstrator in anatomy under Colles and Dease but, after two years, he resigned as he thought the professors were jealous of his succeess with students. The professors thought that Kirby treated them badly by his resignation, as shown in this letter by Colles. "I communicated to my colleague, Mr. Dease, your note of the 15th instant. We regret and are surprised that you should now feel yourself obliged to withdraw from that engagement with us which you entered some weeks ago, when Mr. Garnett waited on you for the purpose of reconciling the differences then existing between you and us. No doubt, we shall be put to some temporary inconvenience by having our arrangements for the season broken up at this late period. These, however, we shall endeavour by suitable exertions, to surmount." It was then that Kirby founded the Peter Street school and he had as large a medical practice as a surgical one. He was president of the Surgeons' College in 1823 and again in 1832, and succeeded Sir Henry March as professor of medicine in the Surgeons' School in 1832, when he closed his private school. Kirby tells us of his hard road to professional success, his work from five in the morning to ten at night and his domestic misfortunes, with his wife dying on the birth of their sixteenth child, leaving him with nine young children to bring up. But to the public Kirby was one of the most ornate "characters" in the Dublin medical scene and naturally was not overlooked by "Erinensis".

"To him the firing of the first gun that announced the passing of the French Army over the heights of Sierra Morena, was music of that agreeable kind, comprising the '*utile dulce*', and the succeeding cannonades, telegraphed from the Isle of Leon, were pregnant with meaning, for he sapiently conjec-

tured that where there was so much noise, it was not too
much to presume that there were some bones broken also,
and that they would of course require surgical assistance.
Besides these manifestations of fortune in his favour abroad,
the Goddess condescended to make known her divine will
at home; as there was shortly after a commission received by
the principal practitioners of the city to send out such of
their pupils as they considered competent to the important
duties of cutting adhesive plaster and attending as nurses
upon the sick. His vision of future success was now no longer
baseless as this confirmation of its correctness placed it upon
a stable foundation. To meet, therefore, this new demand in
the surgical market and to heal the bleeding wounds of his
countrymen, 'a house with back concerns' was hired in Peter
Street, and by a summary process of mechanism, was converted into an anatomical theatre. The establishment
was no sooner fitted up than it was crowded by a motley
audience of every possible shade of character. Apothecaries,
old and young, spurning their lowly association, bade an
eternal adieu to the pestle and their native hamlets, and
committed themselves to be ground at Kirby's Mill. The
class was numerous and soon assembled, but there was still
wanted an appendage to the 'concern' to make it complete,
for the pupils on going to London were required to produce
certificates of attendance at some hospital. A hospital was
therefore added, of dubious character no doubt; but the
form, and not the substance, it seems, was all that was
demanded by the 'examiners' on the other side of the channel.
There was then no '*Lancet*' to set them right, to expose the
evil tendencies of professional chicane, and to unravel the
sophisticated webs of reviewers, whose accommodating creed
consists in the convertibility of truth into falsehood. But to
return—in the celebrated *La Charité* of Peter Street, there was
but one bed and we assure our readers that when we visited
the place there was no bottom in the same. When a case,
however, presented itself, remediable by STEEL, the scat-
tered members of the bed were collected, and if the result of
the operation happened to be favourable, it was made
known in due course through the medium of the morning

journals." . . . "The graceful swing of his chaise, as it plays upon the obedient springs, would learn to be communicated by his own versatile movements, in the solemn rumbling of its wheels, imagination conjures up the awe-inspiring pathos of his oratory, and in the varnished stiffness and profusion of its embellishments, fancy cannot fail to find a similitude for the gaudy tints of his rhetorical tulips. All, indeed, are but parts of one stupendous whole. The very horses, as they toss their heads on high, seem proud of their subjection to so stately a master. The light azure livery and silver lace of the mortal Phaeton, holding the reins, are but the creation of his fertile invention; and the military shoulder knots of a blooming boy, perched like another Ariel upon the box behind, are emblematic of his picturesque taste. The entire equipage looks big with importance and as it flouts your gaze in its rapid motion over the muttering pavements, you should think fortune itself was dragged into captivity at its wheels." . . . "Mr. Kirby, being aware that the persons who composed his audience at one period were intended for military practice, and faithful in the discharge of his duties, took advantage of every expedient to exemplify these cases which they would have to treat. Gun-shot wounds were, of course, a favourite theme; as he happened not to have much experience in the subject, except what he could learn from the misfortune of an occasional duel, he hit upon a very ingenious alternative of making up for the deficiency. It was one of a strange description, to be sure, but quite characteristic of its inventor. For the purpose of demonstrating the destructive effects of fire-arms upon the human frame, Bully's acre* gave up its cleverest treasures for the performance of the experiment. The *subjects*, being placed with military precision along the wall, the lecturer entered with his pistol in his hand, and levelling the mortiferous weapon at the enemy, magnanimously discharged several rounds, each followed by repeated bursts of applause. As soon as the smoke and approbation subsided, then came the tug of war. The wounded were examined, arteries were taken up, bullets were extracted, bones were set, and every spectator

---

*The Hospital Fields burial ground at Kilmainham.

fancied himself on the field of battle, and looked upon Mr.
Kirby as a prodigy of genius and valour for *shooting dead men*.
It is disputed why Mr. Kirby has discontinued the sham
battles. Some say that the return of peace has rendered his
explosions unnecessary, but others, with more truth, affirm
that the memorable pistols with which he was wont to do so
much execution upon the dead, were quietly delivered up by
him to one of the living, as he was returning on a moon-shiny
night in his gig from the country. Oh, what a falling off was
there! The hero of *Peterloo* disarmed by a foot-pad!"

While Colles and the Surgeons' School were flourishing in
those early decades of the nineteenth century and erecting for
themselves that magnificent College we know today, the reader
may well wonder what was happening to the University and
the Physicians in the interval. We saw how Trinity and the
Physicians came together again in 1785 and established by Act
of Parliament a combined school—the School of Physic,
Trinity providing the Regius professor of Physic and professorships in anatomy and chirurgery, botany and chemistry, while
the Physicians nominated King's professors, in the practice of
medicine, institutes of medicine, and materia medica (and later
a King's professorship in midwifery) from Sir Patrick Dun's
estates. All appeared to be settled for the rapid development of
this school, but the very opposite occurred and the Trinity
school reached its nadir in its long history. There were many
reasons for all this happening. George Cleghorn, the respected
professor of anatomy and chirurgery, took ill and died. His
successor and nephew, James Cleghorn, was not of the same
calibre and retired on the grounds of ill health, which he
apparently enjoyed for some twenty years afterwards; to be followed in the chair by William Hartigan, old, good-humoured
and complacent. Then a battle royal raged between Edward
Hill, the Regius professor of Physic and also professor of botany,
and his colleague, Robert Perceval, the professor of chemistry.
Eighteenth century medicine was much closer to letters than
it is now. Hill was one of those brilliant scholars who could
equally well have adorned a chair in English literature. He was
for many years engaged in an edition of Milton's *Paradise Lost*,

though this survives only in manuscript. Perceval had an extensive medical practice, but contributed little to the science of chemistry. His intellectual pursuits were on the higher plane of theology; he published an essay on the Divinity of Jesus Christ in which he maintained that he proved by Scripture texts that Christ, though divine, is distinct from God, who had delegated to him his divine attributes. These two professors were now to be the chief antagonists over the provision of clinical teaching in Dublin. Hill wanted a botanic garden, the *Hortus Sanitatis* or physic garden of the ancients. Perceval wanted a clinical school, as in Edinburgh, and Perceval was to have his way. At first Mercer's Hospital was approached with a view to having clinical lectures there, but this arrangement did not continue for long, as the physicians at Mercer's Hospital were opposed to the scheme (and one of their number had previously been defeated in a King's professorship appointment) and in any case the clinical school was only allotted a "cold garret not fit for the purpose". Then Stephen Dickson, one of the King's professors, decided to have a house in Clarendon Street fitted up as a hospital of seventeen beds, but this scheme fell through in less than two years, as it was financially impossible to continue. Then Perceval took over the leadership of the scheme. He had a house in Blind Quay, now Wellington Quay, fitted up as a hospital in 1797. It also failed after four years, and subscription lists for its support by the public yielded only £96 in that period. Then Mercer's Hospital offered better terms, but Perceval was not interested or sympathetic to any such arrangement. Meanwhile the King's professors, led by Dickson, filed a suit claiming the greater part of Dun's estate as salaries, including two years' arrears. The appeal to the Irish House of Lords in 1796 brought forth this address from the Lord Chancellor. "In my judgment the conduct on the part of the appellants must be considered in a court of equity as a gross and shameless fraud, and whether the letter of this act will bear them out or whether it will not, at any other tribunal, it seems to me to be most perfectly clear that they should be scouted from a court of equity with shame and disgrace." It should be noted that this Lord Chancellor, Lord Clare, was none other than The Right Honourable John Fitzgibbon who, as Attorney General a few years before, had given his opinion unequivocally in favour of their claims. Stephen Dickson now disappeared from the scene, as did some £152 13s. 3d. in library funds entrusted to his care as librarian to the Physicians' College. Perceval decided that Lord Clare was a man to be cultivated and Hill described these overtures by Perceval as "the unnecessary conversations of this restless busybody". A committee of the Irish House of Lords was set up to enquire into the disposal of Sir Patrick Dun's estates. One of the minor disclosures was a hogshead of claret dispensed by the Physicians' president and allegedly paid for from Dun's estate—the hogshead assuming enormous cubic capacity as the committee continued its evidence. The noble Lords decided that Dun's estates should provide £100 per annum for each of the King's professors and the remainder to endow a hospital bearing his name. A new School of Physic Act, 1800, incorporating the committee's decision, was passed by the Irish Parliament—the second last they passed before passing themselves out of office. Perceval who throughout was acting against the interests of the Physicians' College, of which he was a fellow, was later rewarded, as can only happen in Ireland, with the honorary fellowship of that college. There can be little doubt that Perceval was the most able of his contemporaries. Decisions had to be made, but the endowment of a hospital was never the intention of Sir Patrick Dun. Dun's famous will was not to be ended even by the 1800 Act, and it required an act of another Irish Parliament over a century later to dispose of it finally. Perceval in later life suffered considerable pain and disability of his hip joints and considered the lesion to be gout. Colles was consulted and disagreed with the diagnosis, and was later to demonstrate these hip joints following a post mortem examination at the Pathological Society of Dublin showing them to be typical examples of morbus coxae senilis.

Sir Patrick Dun's Hospital was opened for clinical lectures in 1812, although the hospital was not finally completed until 1816. In the interval the few Trinity students that there were received clinical teaching at Dr. Steevens' Hospital under Dr. Crampton and later at the Meath Hospital under Dr. Whitley Stokes. But it was the appointment of James Macartney to the chair of anatomy and chirurgery in 1813 that "made" the Trinity School.

James Macartney was born in Armagh in 1770; his youth had been an unhappy one, and his early education as chequered as that of John Hunter. A premature love affair had turned his thoughts to surgery. "Not," as he wrote, "from any taste of the profession, but in the hope that it would harden my heart, as it did others." Coming to Dublin in 1793 to study at the Surgeons' School, where he was apprenticed to Hartigan, he no doubt met Colles as his fellow student. They were later to be professors in rival medical schools. Then, once more, he fell in love with a Miss Singer, a beautiful girl. "I might," he said, "have proposed to her if she had not been so extraordinarily thin. From the threadbare figure she grew to be one of the most bulky women I ever saw. How little people can tell what their wives may become in person, temper, or principle." Macartney went back later and married his first love. During his student days in Dublin, Macartney appears to have associated with the United Irishmen movement and made friends with all the leaders, including Wolfe Tone; but later as the movement became more militant, he withdrew from its activities. Macartney was now attracted by the reputation of the Great Windmill Street school founded by William Hunter, now continued by Baillie and Cruickshank, and in 1795 he left Dublin, having been released from his apprenticeship by Hartigan. In London his clinical instruction was "now at Guy's, now at Bart's and now at St. Thomas's". He did so well in the anatomy course that, whilst still a student, Abernethy appointed him to a demonstratorship in anatomy at St. Bartholomew's Hospital, and in 1800, on becoming a member of the College of Surgeons in London, he was immediately appointed to a lectureship in comparative anatomy at St. Bartholomew's Hospital the first appointment of its kind in a London hospital school. Macartney directed his attention to surgical or topographical anatomy and aimed to produce a book on the subject, but this, however, did not materialise. Macalister tells us that when demonstrating, and to give his students confidence, Macartney would tie the femoral artery blindfold and, upon occasion, ligated the vessel successfully with his back to the subject.

Difficulties now arose between Macartney and his colleagues at St. Bartholomew's Hospital, which forced him to resign his demonstratorship, although he retained his lectureship. Charles Bell, impressed by Macartney's talent, tried unsuccessfully to attract him to Edinburgh, and wrote—"Macartney is a man of that activity of mind, that expertness in anatomical pursuits, his abilities and industry have been so especially shown in the subject of his lectures, that a regard for science weakens my desire to see him in the present instance successful in his application to obtain the surgeoncy he is seeking." However, Macartney did enter the Army as a surgeon in 1803 and, as he was stationed in the Isle of Wight, he obtained leave each spring to deliver his lectures in London. He resigned his lectureship in 1811, the same year that he was elected to the fellowship of the Royal Society, and in that year also he went to Ireland with his regiment. As the regiment was disembodied in 1812, Macartney decided to remain in Ireland. He was obviously interested in the Trinity chair, now that Hartigan was ill and not expected to lecture again—Samuel Wilmot, meanwhile, acting as his deputy. In May 1812 he took the M.D. degree of St. Andrews University and in June 1813 was appointed to the chair of anatomy and chirurgery at Trinity. Macartney, now forty-three, was to hold this chair for twenty-four "contentious" years. Full of vigour and energy, he was determined from the start to raise the school to the level of the better organised schools of London and Edinburgh. The reformer is rarely popular, and Macartney speedily found the attitude of his new colleagues on the staff to vary from one of sheer indifference to that of active antagonism. The old Anatomy House was in a neglected condition, with less than a hundred ill-mounted and ill-kept preparations, most of which had to be replaced from his own collection. The little dissecting room, with its five tables, had sufficed for Hartigan's dwindling classes, but by the end of his first year Macartney found himself trying to accommodate 116 pupils, each of whom had been drawn to the school by the merit of his teaching—in a room twenty feet square. Compelled to repeat his lectures twice in each day, as he could not trust the flooring to bear the full class at a single sitting, he roundly declared that "there was not a public anatomical institution in Europe so unfit for its purpose as the one in Trinity College". But it was not only the Anatomy House that was in disrepair, the whole central direction of the College and University was, in the words of Sir John Mahaffy, in "its disgraceful forty years".

The reign of Trinity's great eighteenth-century Provosts, Baldwin, the autocrat, Andrews, the man of fashion, Hely-Hutchinson, the politician, ended in 1794 on the death of the latter. The dons, understandably, from their recent experience, did their best to secure an academic or clerical appointment, and supported by Edmund Burke, who declared that "no choice can exist out of the University so good as that which is furnished within its walls", they gained for themselves the principle that the "senior major of the regiment" or the next senior was regularly promoted to the office. Richard Murray, who had been a fellow for forty-five years, was appointed Provost in 1794, but only lived for five years. A kindly old gentleman, he was a mathematician and author of a textbook on logic. We see his name on Abraham Colles' B.A. diploma (1795) and also amongst the Freeman of the city of Dublin. The succeeding Provosts, Kearney (1799–1806), Hall (1806–1811), Elrington (1811–1820), Kyle (1820–1831), were all clerical dons, who used this office to obtain lucrative clerical sees. By a curious coincidence, the influence of Primate Boulter's policy and the exclusion of Irishmen from bishoprics had also passed away, and so we find the Provosts passed on to the episcopal bench, leaving no mark upon the College, and taking no interest in aught beyond the decent management of the routine studies of the place. Mahaffy concludes, "The history of Trinity from the appointment of Murray (1794) to that of Bartholomew Lloyd in 1831 is probably the least creditable in all the three centuries. During these disgraceful forty years no public display brought the College into notice, except the lavish feast for George IV (1821). At the same time, the numbers of students was very great, the income of seniors in renewal fines, and of juniors in tutors' fees, larger than they were ever before or since; yet these were the years which justly earned for the University of Dublin the now obsolete title of the 'Silent Sister'. There was a day when Oxford, for like reasons, had obtained the kindred name of 'The Widow of Sound Learning'."

Macartney first attacked the use of the Latin language in examinations and in lectures. The King's professors disagreed and reported this to their College. By a resolution of the Physicians' College, the King's professors were directed "not to be present at any examinations for medical degrees, in which any question might be put or an answer received in the English language". They also resolved that all the clinical lectures in Sir Patrick Dun's Hospital and reports of the cases taken there were to be in the Latin tongue. The Trinity Board forwarded this resolution to Hill, the Regius professor of Physic. Hill replied as follows: "Examinations in English as introductory to a learned profession are so absolutely contrary to the conceptions which I entertain of a literary education, as to render it impossible that I should tolerate them in any case in which I possessed any influence. No instance of this kind has ever happened to me, and in the examinations of medical candidates under a *liceat ad examinandum*, how could I in any possibility be satisfied thro' such examination of the candidates being *doctrina idoneum*." Next, Macartney was in the habit of performing post-mortem examinations on the patients who had died in Sir Patrick Dun's Hospital. The King's professors objected to this procedure, doubtless feeling that it was not consistent with either their dignity or reputation that their clinical diagnoses should be revised by the post-mortem findings of an unsympathetic colleague. Another difficulty was that the clinical professors could not consult with Macartney even over a hospital case, as he had no licence from the Physicians' College. Four years later they made him an honorary fellow of that college. Dun's Hospital in those days and for many decades later was simply a medical clinic and Macartney's attempt to have a surgical ward was negatived by physicians. These King's professors only used the hospital during the university term, and the hospital found it necessary to appoint a physician to carry on the normal running of the hospital at other times. In 1827 Dr. Jonathan Osborne was appointed physician-in-ordinary to the hospital. There was nothing "ordinary" about the directions in Osborne's will. Being long afflicted with rheumatism, he requested that he should be buried in the upright position as "he did not want any fellow at the Resurrection to have an advantage over him"! And buried upright he was.

Back at Trinity, Macartney, after many years of struggle with the College Board, finally had a new Anatomy House erected in 1825, and declared at the opening ceremony that "it was more valuable a gift upon the community by building this House than if they had founded ten hospitals". Colles and Macartney afford a fascinating study in contrasts. Both received their first lessons in anatomy from Hartigan in the old Mercer Street school and now, working side by side in one small city during the twenty-three years in which the respective tenures of their chairs overlapped, we have no record of their ever having met, and while the posthumous reputation of Colles is world wide, the name of Macartney is virtually forgotten today, even in the Trinity school to which he gave the best years of his life to raise it to its heights. "From first to last Colles was the surgeon-anatomist, and his approach to anatomy was that of the practical surgeon who, so far from regarding it as an independent discipline, constantly explained its sub-serviency to the operator's needs. Colles was the accurate observer of all that passed before his eyes, but was 'cautious to a fault' in drawing conclusions from what he had seen. Macartney, the unlettered apprentice, may no less accurately be described as the anatomist-surgeon. His was the more enquiring intelligence of the two. Macalister's assertion that he was the most philosophical surgeon that his generation had produced in Ireland seems well supported by the quality of his published work. During his years with Mathew Baillie at the Great Windmill Street school, he had absorbed some share of the Hunterian curiosity as to the inter-relationship of all animate things" (Doolin).

At the Surgeons' School, as at Dr. Steevens' Hospital, Colles was the accepted leader, a quiet, modest, good-tempered man, on easy terms with students and colleagues alike. The Surgeons' School was young and vigorous, the child of a new century, its traditions yet to make, with all who worked therein fired with the firm intention of making good. Macartney, like all great reformers, was bound to meet with some unpopularity, but seems rather to have looked for it than avoided it. We must, however, remember that his period in the chair was in the midst of Trinity's "disgraceful forty years". Trinity being moulded largely on the model of Cambridge, its medical school as yet almost untouched by the modern spirit, the surgeon was *persona non grata*, his craft still regarded as a form of manual labour, unworthy of the consideration of a King's professor. For twenty-four years of unbroken contention, Macartney *was* the Trinity School. Macartney resigned his chair in 1837, following an impossible row with his College and his colleagues, having previously sold the contents of his museum to Cambridge for an annuity of £100 a year for ten years. He died in March, 1843, some nine months before Colles. The last words he wrote may form his epitaph:

> "The last great event is the extinction of the systematic functions which is commonly called death. As soon as the vitality of the tissue is lost, the body becomes subject to the laws of inorganic matter. The greater part of it is exhaled and is carried by the winds and clouds to distant regions, and finally they descend with rains to fertilise the earth. We thus repay our great debt to nature, and return the elements of our bodies to the common storehouse. Thus ends this strange eventful history.
>
> > All forms that perish, other forms supply:
> > (By turns we catch the vital breath and die),
> > Like bubbles on the sea of matter borne,
> > They rise, they break, and to that sea return."

CHAPTER 7

The Colles Publications

Abraham Colles published three books and a dozen surgical papers (see Appendix). Several papers from his manuscripts were later edited and published (1853–1857) after his death by his son William, as were also his lectures on surgery by Simon McCoy (1844).

His first publication, a *Treatise on Surgical Anatomy*, 1811, is perhaps of most interest to surgeons. This little slim volume was intended to be a part of a major work, which however was not completed. Approximately half of this work is devoted to the anatomy of hernia, then follow brief chapters on the anatomy of the abdomen, neck and throat, thorax, pelvis, bladder, external genitalia and perineum, and finally, chapters on the passage of the catheter and lithotomy. The work is prefaced by an address to the pupils of his College, a few excerpts of which are given below.

"It requires but little to prove that to form a good surgeon, a good education is the first and most essential requisite. For nothing contributes more effectually either to expand the understanding or to mature the judgment, than an early exercise of the intellectual faculties. It enables the student to take more clear and comprehensive views of the facts which occur to his observation. It teaches him to deduce from those facts none but logical inferences, and secures his reason from the danger of being hurried away by the speciousness of false analogies . . . ."

"On the necessity of classical information, it is needless to dwell, because in fact no person can be admitted a registered pupil of the College of Surgeons until he has undergone a public examination in Latin and Greek, before the court of examiners; but as the course appointed to be read for entrance comprises little more than Virgil, Sallust and Horace in one

language, and Lucian, Xenophon and Homer in the other,
I would recommend it to you occasionally to refresh and
extend your knowledge of the classics at your leisure hours.
A knowledge of French is scarcely less necessary than that of
Greek and Latin, for many of the most eminent works on
surgical subjects have been published originally in that
language, and have not yet been translated into our own;
and fortunately for us, the study of French is one which requires neither much time nor labour. A slight application
for a few months will enable you to read any surgical author
in this language, with sufficient facility . . . ."

"But, besides a knowledge of the classics, an acquaintance
with the sciences also is necessary to complete the preparatory
education of the surgeon . . . . no science tends so effectually
to strengthen the understanding and to improve the reasoning faculties as that of mathematics, for it requires that
complete retirement of the mind within itself, that straight-
forward, unbroken progress of thought, which can alone
enable us to follow up a long chain of arguments and arrive
at a remote conclusion . . . . it is also in a great degree the key
to most of the other sciences . . . ."

    "Natural philosophy will be found of great use to explain
some of the functions of the animal body and the laws to
which they are subject . . . . you should, however be careful
to apply them with the utmost caution. You should recollect
that in the animal system physical laws are often counter-
acted by the superior powers of the living principle. From an
inattention to this fact originated most of the errors in
physiology and pathology into which the great Boerhaave
was betrayed. It was owing to this that he conceived the
circulation of the blood through the arterial and venous
systems to be subject to the same laws which regulate the
motions of fluids through inanimate tubes. A theory which,
though perfectly consonant to the laws of hydraulics, is
yet totally incompatible with the laws of the living system.
On these misapplied principles did he also account for the
derangements which take place in the circulation from
disease, and on this fundamental error is built his celebrated
theory of inflammation . . . ."

"Chemistry, gentlemen, affords such a luminous explanation of the great phenomena of nature, and leads to such important improvements in the various arts subservient to human life that mankind at large must regard it as a science at once most pleasing and most eminently useful. To the surgical student in particular, it is of indispensable importance. For without the knowledge of the chemical properties of those substances which he uses in the composition of external applications, or of internal remedies, how is it possible for him to avoid combining together medicines which, though innocent or useful in themselves, may yet by their combination be rendered either dangerously active or totally inert? .... But the advantages which the surgeon derives from the knowledge of chemistry are not confined to the composition and administrations of medicine. This science is of still more material use to him in elucidating several important phenomena of the animal economy; for by chemical analysis we acquire a more accurate knowledge of the component parts of many substances which are secreted from the general mass of the blood and lodged in various cavities of the body. Thus we learn more clearly the composition of urine and bile, and thus we gain a more distinct idea of certain morbid changes which take place in these fluids, and in the formation of biliary and urinary calculi .... I well know how fashionable it is to lavish on chemistry the most unqualified praise, and to attribute to it the most unbounded utility to the study and practice of medicine; but however popular the study of this fascinating science may be, however ardent the hopes and enthusiastic the expectations of its admirers, I trust that I shall be able to satisfy your ingenious and unprejudiced minds that the vital properties of the human system depend not on its chemical principles, and that the great and complicated operations of the animal economy are not subject to the same laws that govern the minute detached particules of inanimate matter ...."

"So inseparably connected are the two sciences of medicine and surgery that he who hopes to practice either profession with benefit to his patient or confidence in himself, must take care to combine the study of both .... Let it not be

supposed that I will inculcate the idea of unnecessarily
uniting the practice of both physic and surgery in the same
person; on the contrary, I am decidedly of opinion that in
great cities the surgeon should never undertake the care of a
case purely medical, nor the physician of a case purely
surgical. All I mean to assert is that the study of both professions should be combined by the man who wishes to practise either to the greatest advantage. But this knowledge
once acquired, the practitioner should direct his attention to
one branch only . . . ."

"Among all those sciences which are subservient to the
profession of surgery, anatomy justly claims the first and
highest rank; it is not only of the greatest importance, but
of the most indispensable necessity both to the study and
practice of surgery. It is in fact the very basis of all surgical
education, the only foundation on which a solid superstructure
can be raised. But it is much to be lamented that the very
science which, of all your professional studies, is the most
important and indispensable, should be at the same time
beyond all comprehension the most difficult and disgusting.
It is greatly regretted that the student should find it so hard
to acquire a knowledge of anatomy, and the practitioner
should so soon lose that anatomical knowledge which has
cost him so much time and labour to acquire . . . . In the first
place, the authors of all elementary systems of anatomy describe the various parts of the human frame as if of equal
importance, instead of giving to each part just that degree
of attention it deserves, and no more. Thus they are as full
and circumstantial in their description of the minute rami-
fications of an artery or nerve, as in that of the trunk or
principal branches; by these means the mind is over-crowded
by the collection of so much superfluous matter, and the
memory over-burdened by the pressure of so much dead
weight. The language, too, in which these descriptions are
conveyed is no less tedious than the descriptions themselves
are trifling. By labouring after a minute and unattainable
accuracy, it serves only to impress an idea of difficulty, when
no difficulty really exists. Another essential mistake is that
of considering anatomy in no other light than as a science in

itself, distinct and independent of any other; instead of considering it as a science altogether subservient to the practice of medicine and surgery. Hence the inexperienced student, taught to regard anatomy without any reference to its uses, views it only as a collection of detached and uninteresting facts, and a catalogue of barbarous and unmeaning terms. Whereas, had he in every step of his progress been shown the connection between the anatomical structures of each part and the surgical diseases and operations to which it is subject, he would have had such a lively interest exited in his mind, as must have compelled him to overcome the natural difficulties of the study, and must have fixed in his memory the indelible impression of the structure of the parts . . . . . Anatomists divided this science into several distinct branches as osteology, myology, neurology, etc. corresponding to the different distinct parts of the animal frame. These divisions they term systems. Each system they describe separately, without taking any notice in the descriptions of its connections with other systems, unless where it happened that that which was the immediate subject of the examination, should have remained absolutely unintelligible without such a reference. And succeeding anatomists have since continued to tread implicitly in the footsteps of their predecessors. By these means, we are certainly enabled to examine the several parts with an accuracy and to describe them with a precision before unknown. But though the description of each particular part be now more perfect, yet the plan is still so far defective, that the description of any one part seldom reminds the student of any other, the examination of any one system seldom leads him to trace its connections and relations with other systems, nor do many detached views of the several parts enable him to take any general and connected view of the whole . . . . In fact, the student who has been employed in acquiring anatomical knowledge of the different divisions or systems of the human body, has but encountered all the difficulties without securing any of the benefits. The study of anatomy, too, generally ends at that period where it begins to be useful. To supply that defect for the pupils of this School is the design of the present work.''

In his paper *On the operation of tying the subclavian artery*
(1815), Colles tells us that shortly after his appointment to
the College chairs, he directed his attention to the study of the
subclavian artery, with a view to tying the vessel for distal
aneurysm. John Bell's description of the anastomosing vessels
about the shoulder joint encouraged Colles to hope for its final
success.

> "Still, however, I did not feel justified in stating any opinion
> to the pupils of the College, for as yet the operation had not
> only been untried in practice, but the proposal wanted even
> the sanction of analogy. Then Mr. Abernethy (1797) gave
> the world his first account of the operation of tying the
> external iliac artery. From this moment I felt myself author-
> ised openly to express my sentiments, and every year since I
> have occasion, both in the anatomical and surgical course,
> not only to state to the class my sentiments generally on the
> subject, but to point out to them the manner in which I
> conceived the operation might be performed. A case of
> axillary aneurysm having, in the year 1809, come under my
> care in the hospital, I proposed this operation, on which
> I had so long meditated, to the other surgeons in consultation.
> The proposal, however, was over-ruled, chiefly on the grounds
> of the operation never having been performed, and I confess
> that I yielded to the voice of the majority with the less
> reluctance, because I felt a secret apprehension of some
> terrible revolution being produced in the frame by tying an
> artery of such magnitude close to the heart. This patient,
> in a few months, fell victim to the disease, but neither by argu-
> ment, nor influence, nor stratagem, could I obtain an
> opportunity of examining the body."

In 1811 Ramsden published his case of ligation of the subclavian
artery, although the operation was unsuccessful. In 1811 and
again in 1813, Colles tied the right subclavian artery for
aneurysm, but both cases died later from sepsis. The operations
were extremely difficult on account of the extent and site of
the lesions, and were formidable procedures in the conscious
patient. Colles concludes: "Although this operation has not yet
proved ultimately successful, yet I think we should not despair

The history of surgery furnishes parallel instances of operations, now generally adopted, which, in the first few trials, failed of success." In 1820 Robert Liston performed the first successful operation in Britain of ligation of the subclavian artery, and in that operation he used as retractors the flexible copper (prince's metal) spatulas introduced by Colles; and so highly did he appreciate these simple instruments that he wrote: "I consider them as the greatest addition made to our surgical instruments for many years." In 1822 Charles H. Todd, Colles' co-professor, successfully tied the subclavian artery at the Richmond Hospital, Dublin. It has often been stated that Colles tied the innominate artery and was the first surgeon to do so. This statement is almost certainly untrue, and the writer is satisfied that no such record exists. Possibly the exposure and opening of the sheath of that major vessel during the ligation of the first stage of the right subclavian artery has led to this misstatement.

In 1817, Colles published an interesting paper on *The Distortion termed Varus or Club Feet*. He preferred treatment of infants, and after trial of the methods then in use, which he found unsatisfactory, he evolved a light and simple apparatus which might be applied to an infant not more than a fortnight old, and never failed to accomplish the cure of the worst cases within a space of three months. The apparatus illustrated consisted of a shoe made of chamois leather doubled, and having between its two layers a sole of strong tin interposed. The tin is cut to the size of the sole of the foot, having, however, two small projections left, one opposite the ball of the great toe, and the other opposite the other ankle. Each of these projections has a longitudinal slit, designed to receive the shouldered end of a splint. After a very clear description of this splint and minute details of its use and management, Colles continues:

"That this deformity has been repeatedly cured by other and very different plans, I make not the smallest doubt; but still I think the plan here recommended will be found to deserve a preference, when it is considered that it combines the following advantages. First, the apparatus is so simple, that instead of requiring an ingenious artist to construct it, it can be made by such common tradesmen as can be found in every country town or village. Secondly, the expense of it is so very trifling as not to require more than a few shillings to provide all that may be necessary for completing the cure of any individual case. Thirdly, the application of it is attended with very little trouble, the apparatus not requiring to be adjusted oftener than every fourth or sixth day. And, lastly, this plan of treatment effects the most complete cure in a very short time, and without being productive of any pain or uneasiness to the child, restoring the limb to the most perfect shape, and ensuring to it the most free and ample power of motion. But though the subjects of this malady may be hereafter relieved in the first stage of infancy, yet the present race of unfortunate sufferers, who have outgrown this favourable period, still retain every claim to our care. Anxious to ascertain if the apparatus which succeeded so well in one case, would succeed in the other, I tried one of similar form, but of much greater strength, for the cure of patients from three to twelve years of age. But I am sorry to say that I had by no means the same success with children as I had with infants. In fact this apparatus was much less efficient in cases of long standing than the apparatus recommended by Professor Scarpa. It is highly probable, that the instrument which Scarpa describes may be found, in many instances, entitled to the encomiums he bestows on it; in many other instances I fear it may disappoint our expectations, as it will be found to require a much greater length of time than he considers necessary to expect a cure. For I apprehend that there are not only different degrees but different kinds of this deformity, and I am convinced that even the bones themselves, by being long held or exercised in an unnatural position, will become distorted and misshapen, although I am aware that these opinions are contrary to those of Professor Scarpa."

In a paper (1817) on *Trismus Nascentium*, Colles mentions the various conjectures then in vogue as to its cause and the occasional reference to umbilical cord inflammation, without any satisfactory proof in support of the latter opinion. Colles studied the problem for some five years and every year carried out dissections on three or more subjects. He found that the symptoms of the disease in infants closely resembles that of trismus traumaticus of adults. He observed "its occurrence to be confined to the period of separation of the cord, and the healing of the surface from which it is detached, as we observe the trismus traumaticus of adults to occur generally in the sloughing stage of wounds; sometimes when the wound has advanced much further to cicatrization; and very rarely, if ever, do we find either disease coming on after the ulcerated parts are perfectly healed. Another striking correspondence between these diseases is that in general the most severe and rapidly fatal cases of each take place before the fifth day from the date of the wound or birth of the child; and that these cases which occur when the surfaces have made considerable advancement towards healing, are very mild in their symptoms and very slow in their progress. Dissection showed that the skin edges are more raised than normal, the umbilical fossa contained a knob or large papilla, with all the surrounds formed by suppurative inflammation, and the orifice of the umbilical vein was involved". On extending his dissections into the abdomen he found the peritoneum vascular as if from inflammation which had extended upwards to the liver fissure, and similar appearances around the arteries and urachus below. He found the interior of the vein free from inflammation, although its walls were involved and very much thickened; and similar appearances were present in the walls of the arteries. He found these changes in all the cases he examined and never saw them in infants of the same age who had died of other diseases. Colles found the disease more prevalent in children born in the Lying-in Hospital than those born in private houses. He suggested spirits of turpentine as a dressing in the prevention of infection. Labatt, who was then Master of the Lying-in Hospital (Rotunda), however, did not agree with Colles' findings.

In a short paper (1818) Colles describes *A disease of the lymphatic glands of the groin attended with peculiar symptoms.*

"The glandular enlargement, from its progress as well as its situation, was liable to be mistaken for venereal or scrofulous affection. The lower inguinal group are those commonly involved, and the onset of the condition is very insidious, with no skin changes and minimal pain and discomfort only on walking or exertion. The progress of the tumour to suppuration is uniform, though slow, the skin becomes red but not pointed, and the matter is spontaneously discharged at a period varying from the fifth to the eighth week. The cavity of abscess is small in proportion to the extent and hardness of the tumour. The matter is, in general, of a tolerably good consistence; not infrequently a second and sometimes even a third collection of matter forms in the neighbourhood of the first, the tumours exhibiting the same indolent character. The openings by which the matter escapes are narrow and spread not to a large size, preserving rather the appearance of fistulous orifices than degenerating into broad ulcers. In general, they heal spontaneously in the course of two or three months from the period of ulceration . . . . A striking feature of this disease is the trifling degree of pain which attends it. The patients suffer so very little as to be capable of walking about without perceptible lameness. The disease usually occurs in men between the ages of twenty and forty, but in general nearer to the former than to the latter period of life. The patient is affected with headache, which is more severe in the morning, which is increased by stooping. He also admits, when questioned, that he feels more fatigued than usual from long, continued or violent exercise; his pulse is quick, being in no case, when he is out of bed, under 100, and generally beating 120 to the minute. The quickness of the pulse appears the more extraordinary, as it is obviously not produced by a high degree of pain, nor is it accompanied by any discoverable derangement of any other of the functions; on the contrary, the countenance is natural, respiration easy, the skin of temperate heat and not very dry, the tongue clean, the appetite as good as usual, and scarcely ever nocturnal sweats. The patient, however, feels himself more comfortable in the open air than when confined to the house. I have had the opportunity of examining one patient only, while lying in bed in the morning: his pulse was then only 72, but when rising and dressing himself it rose to 110.

The tumour at that time was as large as half a hen's egg and the integuments were not discoloured."

Lees, in a fresh assessment of this paper made with special regard to the knowledge available at that time, writes—"I consider Colles wrote a clear clinical description of what is now known almost universally as *lymphogranuloma inguinale*. He noted-severe headache and a rapid pulse often continued for several weeks. This is not a conspicuous feature of the disease as we now know it, though metastatic and constitutional effects occur occasionally. He recognised that the condition was not syphilis or tuberculosis, and so gets credit for an original observation and wise advice on the treatment of the condition."

With the publication in 1837 of his book, *Practical observations on the venereal disease and on the use of mercury*, Colles was established as one of the great authorities in this field. Some maintain that it was his greatest work. Surgeons had for centuries the care of the "venereal" and there were many and extreme views on its nature. It cannot be a matter of surprise that opinions were divided and treatment wavering and uncertain. One French surgeon announced to the world that there was no such disease as venereal at all! Others regarded "syphilis" as a generic term under which may be classed a number of species, each in itself distinct and separate; each primary sore followed by its own proper and peculiar train of secondary affections, from which there neither is nor can be any deviation. And again there were syphilists who thought not only every sore on the genitals of a particular appearance as venereal, but even held that if a man constitutionally tainted, should happen to receive a cut on the finger or wound in the head, the consequent sore would assume the character of the disease and the matter separated by it become capable of being the medium of contamination. Even in that age (1837) the authority of John Hunter still prevailed and few dared to question his dogmatic writings on the venereal (1786). Hunter drew no distinction between gonorrhoea and syphilis, and did not recognize the infective nature of the secondary stage of syphilis. Hunter's description of the hard chancre as the commonest presentation of the primary lesion was incorrect, as was his denial that a chancre could occur in the urethra. Some of Hunter's errors were corrected by Benjamin Bell, and Colles was to correct others, in a work in which he paid glowing tributes to the genius of Hunter, "whose invaluable treatise poured a flood of light not only on the natural history of this disease, but also on its pathology and treatment". It is remarkable that all these men, and many others, by their own observations contributed so much to the elucidation of that strange disease. Another century was to dawn before the Egyptian darkness was to disappear in the light of the discovery of the causal micro-organism, *Treponema Pallidum*, by Schaudinn and Hoffman in 1905, and Wasserman's complement fixation test a year later.

Mercury, on account of its wonderful therapeutic and physical properties, had long attracted the attention of both chemists and medical men. The chemists had endowed it with almost human attributes, and considered that it possessed the properties of metals and non-metals. Mercury is mentioned by Theophrastus in 315 B.C. and is believed to have been long before that time used medicinally in both India and China. Dioscorides gave it the name of hydrargyrum, or water of silver, and it was also known as the 'proteus of nature', 'the fugitive salt' ,and 'the mineral spirit'. For many centuries it was used in the treatment of syphilis, and both Hunter and Colles regarded it as "specific" for this disease. In medicine the drug was used both externally in the form of ointments, plasters, and fumigations, and internally not only as crude quicksilver, but also in the form of various salts. Huge doses were given and the efficacy of the treatment was estimated by the quantity of the salivation produced. Boerhaave is said to have taught "that if the patient spits three pints or two quarts in the twenty-four hours it is sufficient, but that, if he spits less, more mercury must be given". In Dr. Steevens' Hospital there were for many years large pewter mugs for the patients to spit into, and the efficacy of the mercurial treatment was measured by the number of these mugs that the patient could fill with saliva in the day. These mugs were used in the hospital for many years during the nineteenth century, but unfortunately not one is now to be found. In 1740, the hospital proposed fitting up one of their houses in Bow Lane as a centre for salivating patients, but this scheme was not proceeded with. In 1757, the hospital fitted up proper salivating wards in the hospital. In Dublin, also, there were certain lodging houses frequented by the "young bucks" for the salivation courses. In London, Hutchinson betrayed a professional vexation at the number of wealthy young Englishmen who went to Aix-la-Chapelle for the "rubbings", when such treatment was equally available at home. The "fluxing" or "salivating" of a patient was always regarded as a serious matter in the special wards provided in the hospital. The patient was to be bled from the arm, to the quantity of some 12 ounces, "in order to attenuate the blood so that there might be room for it after it is rarefied by the mercury." The patient was also to be purged "lest intestinal commotions should be raised at the same time as the salivation". In addition to this the patient was to bathe for an hour every morning and evening, if he was strong, but if weakly once a day. In either case the stomach was to be empty at the time the bath was taken. The number of baths varied according to the constitution of the patient, but each morning in the bath or in bed, the patient was to take "a draught of clarified chalybeated whey, turned with an infusion of gerimander, watercresses, chervil, etc., or broth made of chicken, or a piece of veal, boiled with diluting, cooling, vulnerary herbs, such as wild savory, saxifrage, agrimony, spleenwort, maidenhair, watercresses, etc." When the salivation was well established, bleeding and purging were still employed, and the clothes wherewith the patient was covered during the time of the friction were to be taken off. Great care was to be taken throughout the whole process to prevent the patients taking cold. This traditional regimen was successfully attacked and revolutionised by Hunter with his characteristic bluntness and honesty. "The manner of living under a mercurial course need not be altered from the common, because mercury has no action upon the disease which is more favoured by any one way of life than another. Let me ask anyone what effect eating a hearty dinner and drinking a bottle of wine can have over the action of mercury upon a venereal sore, either to make it affect any part sensibly as falling upon the glands of the mouth, or prevent its effect upon the venereal irritation? In short, I do not see why mercury should not cure the venereal disease under any mode whatsoever of regimen or diet." Colles also cut out the frills of the regimen, although he continued with bloodletting and purgatives—the shades of Gregory were still evident!

There were three methods of administering mercury to "raise a salivation". In the first method, mercury was administered by mouth. A favourite preparation was corrosive sublimate, the active principle of the "catholicon" of Paracelsus, and also of the solution recommended by Van Swieten. Colles favoured a mixture of calomel and lime—the well-known "black wash". The second method was by "unction" or the rubbing into the skin of mercurial ointment—a preparation known as the "Neopolitan ointment" was often used for this purpose. In preparing this ointment the purest mercury revived from cinnebar was to be used. The mercury was to be killed with a sufficient quantity of turpentine in a mortar till reduced to a black powder. To this powder an equal quantity of fresh hog's lard was added, and the ingredients were well rubbed together with a pestle until the particles of the mercury powder were so small as to be invisible. Some preferred to kill the mercury with spittle rather than with turpentine, which often caused skin irritation. The patient was to stand before a good fire and the part of the body to which the ointment was to be applied was to be rubbed with the dry hand till it became red. On the first day ten drachms of ointment were to be rubbed into the feet as far as the ankles. The second rubbing was from the ankles to the knees, and the third from the knees to the buttocks. Then rubbing was to be made on alternate days, so as to be completed on the fifth day. If no salivation was produced on the seventh day, a fourth rubbing was to be made from the buttocks to the loins, and so on to the shoulders and down the arms. Usually three rubbings were enough, and a satisfactory ptyalism was the spitting up from three to six pints in twenty-four hours. "If the discharge is less than three pints it is too small and not sufficient to conquer the disease. If it exceeds the bounds of six pints it will be too violent to be borne by the patient for a sufficient time to get the better of the distemper." When professional rubbers were employed they used pigs' bladders as gloves to protect their hands. The third method of mercurial therapy was by stoving or fumigation. For this one was "to take cinnebar, one ounce, storax, myrrh, olibanum Benjamin, of each half an ounce, mastik, mace, of each two drachms, turpentine which suffices; throw this on coals and let the patient receive it cover'd". This though acknowledged to be very efficacious, was looked upon as a most dangerous method. Colles modified this rather crude method and his cinnebar candles were long in use in Dublin for the local treatment of ulcers. Fumigations normally failed to excite ptyalism, except when the fumes escaped into the mouth, and of course in those cases where the method was used directly for the treatment of mouth and throat ulceration.

The minor complications of the mercurial course were mercurial fever, the development of a rash—*erythema mercuriale*, and a peculiar tendency to corpulency on the termination of the course. But the most serious complication was overdosage, and Colles gives a graphic clinical description of what we would now term mercurial poisoning.

"In some of these cases, however, we find that these alarmingly large doses of mercury do excite a ptyalism, not that gentle, manageable kind which is our anxious wish to obtain, but rather a sudden, a violent, and an ungovernable action which overwhelms the system and threatens destruction to life. The day preceding the appearance of this violent salivation the patient announces its approach by informing us that he was feverish and restless the preceding night, and that he has great headaches or tormina, or dysenteric dejections from his bowels. On the following day his cheeks and lips are enormously swollen, there is a copious and incessant flow of saliva, the tongue is protruded and swollen, the speech is impaired, and deglutition is so impeded that he cannot even drink without much difficulty. Haemorrhages from the gums to a pretty large amount in many instances occur repeatedly; the tongue continuing swollen and protruded, its edges more particularly on their lower surface, become indented and ulcerated from the pressure of the teeth. When awake he hangs his head over some vessel to receive the saliva, which flows copiously and incessantly, and when overcome by fatigue he attempts to sleep, the saliva still flows, and bathes his pillow with a foetid moisture; his sleep is broken and unrefreshing, and is frequently interrupted by a sudden and alarming sense of suffocation, induced partly by the swelling of all the salivary and mucous structures about the mouth and fauces, and partly by the accumulation of the viscid saliva which he is unable to swallow. After two or three weeks passed in this way, but with little alteration, the saliva at length becomes more thick and ropy, and the swelling of the face, tongue and fauces subsides and the patient feels a strong desire for food, but is totally unable to take any in a solid form, and he suffers exquisitely in attempting to swallow any, even the blandest fluid; and thus he is harassed on the one hand by a craving for food and nourishment, and on the other by the apprehension of acute pain attending every attempt at mastication or deglutition. At length, however, the swelling subsides, the ulcers of the mouth heal, and a general improvement in the health occurs; yet even then he often has to lament the continuance of some of the various and serious effects which the excess of mercurial action seldom fails to excite, such as loosening of the teeth, pain and even caries and exfoliation of the alveoli, or of the jaw bone; sometimes the tongue contracts, adhesions to the teeth etc. etc. It will naturally occur now to enquire, can the patient be assured, as some recompense for all the sufferings he has undergone, that the disease for which the mercury has been administered is cured? In many cases this benefit has been gained, though doubtless dearly purchased; but in many other instances, the surgeon as well as the patient observes with regret, and even with dismay, that although the chancre has nearly healed, yet during the last few days it has remained stationary, and also that there is more surrounding hardness than is consistent with the healthy action in the part. It would be needless to comment on the judgement or the feelings of that practitioner who could, under such circumstances, recommend the patient to resume the use of mercury."

Many of these tragedies followed on Hunter's rule that "the quantity of mercury to be thrown into the constitution for the cure of any venereal complaint must be proportioned to the violence of the disease". Colles maintained that the full effect of mercury as a therapeutic measure could be established by minute doses built up with ptyalism acting as a guide. This was his thesis and his teaching, which was the product of his extensive experience and his undoubted talent for observation.

About that time the use of mercury as the traditional treatment for syphilis came to be questioned, and especially whether it was to continue to be regarded as "specific" for the disease, as Hunter and Colles believed it to be. Experiences of British Army surgeons in the Peninsular War, Devergie of France, Oppenheim of Germany and Carmichael of Dublin, to mention but a few, led to the establishment of the "non-mercurial" school. Richard Carmichael, surgeon to the Richmond Hospital, Dublin and respected contemporary, was now to review Colles' book, which he did without a trace of acrimony. "I know how strongly he is wedded to early opinions and associations, and that I might as well attempt to shake a pious Mussulman from his faith, that there is no God but Allah, and that Mahomed is his prophet, as to endeavour to dissuade my friend from his belief in the infallible powers of mercury over every form and every stage of venereal complaints—a belief which may aptly be parodied by a doctrine, the orthodoxy of which he will not dispute, that to overcome the malady there is no God but mercury, and Abraham is his prophet!" Colles and Carmichael knew that they were working in the dark, and "dark ground illumination" was still a long way off. Colles was quite satisfied that syphilis was a highly infectious and contagious disorder, but of the nature of the infection he had no clearer idea than that it was "a poison". He tells us that "in remote parts of Ireland, the poor people are so strongly impressed with the notion of the very infectious nature of venereal disease, that if they be told that a stranger whom they had lodged in their home for a night had this disease, they would instantly burn the straw seat upon which he had been sitting". Though Colles did not know the nature of the infection he had clear ideas of the usual method in which it was transmitted. He had been told that infection resulted from "sitting on a public privy", but he had never been satisfied with the truth of the statement, and adds that Mr. Obré held similar views. Obré had been for many years extensively engaged in treating the venereal disease, and when Colles asked him if he believed that the disease was ever propagated in this manner, Obré shrewdly answered, "that it was sometimes the manner in which *married* men contracted it, but *unmarried* men never caught it in this manner"!

Colles' *Lectures on the theory and practice of Surgery* (1844) were edited and published after his death by his pupil Simon McCoy. This publication was not intended as a textbook of surgery, but rather as a record and memento for the thousands of students who had attended Colles' classes in the Surgeons' School. In language, too, the lectures were simple and fluent, and more of a conversational character than the didactic lessons of a teacher. We must of course assess their content in the light of the surgical knowledge available at that time. The professor of surgery of today might also like to be reminded that Colles lectured to a class of two hundred and fifty students at 3 o'clock on Saturday afternoons! Of the forty-nine lectures in the surgical course, ten were on the venereal. A few excerpts from these lectures are given below:

> *Inflammation* was not understood. Its main treatment was by bloodletting—"to make an impression on the system". "Blood was to be withdrawn rapidly to produce fainting, and this must not be from the sight of the lancet, it must be from the detraction of blood and not from the patient's timidity."

> An *Abscess* was healthy and contains simple, healthy pus! Hectic fever, contrary to the views of Cullen and others, was not always due to the presence of pus! "There does not seem to be anything in the qualities of simple, healthy pus that would lead us to think it ought to cause so serious an effect on the constitution; it is a mild, bland, semi-fluid secretion, unirritating, tardily yielding to putrefaction, sometimes lying quietly encysted for months in the body, and for years continuing to be secreted from the surfaces of an issue or

ulcer without prejudice to the parts with which it has been in contact. We are still in the dark as to its uses, but, except from circumstances wholly unconnected with its particular nature, we see no injurious effects from its presence." It is interesting to note that Dr. Gregory used to relieve night sweats in his patients by prescribing a meat dinner and a pint of draught porter before their going to bed. Colles was not keen on poultices for inflammation, but if used, he thought the carrot poultice was best.

Erysipelas—"The question has been stated whether this be contagious or not, and it has been adduced in proof to the affirmative that several people in the same ward of a hospital will be attacked with it at the same time, without any obvious cause, and where there is no want of cleanliness and care, but this is only a proof that there is some general predisposing cause with which we are not acquainted, operating in the case. The greatest number of cases occurring in Ireland at the same time, have been remarked to be during the prevalence of very warm, moist weather. Those who believe in fevers being contagious may by the same train of reasoning believe erysipelas so too. It is certainly remarkable that a number of cases will appear at the same time in a hospital in an unaccountable manner, and surgeons at such a time will delay performing any operation that can be delayed for days and months, knowing the great risk the patient will be in getting erysipelas from their incisions. Dr. Harvey of Dr. Steevens' Hospital remembered that there was never an epidemic fever in Ireland that was not followed by numerous cases of erysipelas in the hospital wards."

Tetanus. "Larrey recommended cutting off the wounded limb. I saw my colleague Obré amputate a limb for compound subluxation of the thumb which developed tetanus, but he might as well have left it on!" "I recollect when Dr. Hamilton's book came out it was expected that every disease could be cured by purgatives, and of course they were tried in tetanus; but I found patients died sooner under the treatment than where nothing of the kind was tried . . . ." "I consider oil of turpentine best for wound dressings."

Breast Abscess. "The treatment of these should be almost entirely constitutional, even when the abscess feels ripe it is much better not to open it, except indeed the matter be just under the cuticle, when you just puncture it with a lancet and let out the matter, but in general you ought to avoid a lancet in these cases, for if there be any life or thickness in the parts you cut through, you will excite fresh inflammation and greatly increase the chances of other abscesses developing."

Paronychia. "The third or malignant type is the most serious as the tendon sheath is involved. You must make deep and long incisions down to the bone—you must feel the knife grating on the very bone—you must never tell the patient he is well until the sloughing tendon is thrown out."

Head injury. "When a man gets this injury some will think they cannot be half busy enough and will blister and bleed him and so forth. In fact, the patient's friends, and often the surgeon himself, think that when they see a person in this state, too much cannot be done to bring him out of it, but time must be given for the brain to recover itself, and when one in this state makes any approach towards recovery, in nine cases out of ten, or at least five out of seven, that recovery will be progressive. You must keep the patient on a low diet, but do not precipitate or over zealously do too much or repeat your evacuations too quickly, when you find the symptoms begin to yield—that is when consciousness begins to return, when he ceases to pass his urine and faeces involuntarily, etc."

Depressed fracture of the skull. "Should a patient with a slightly depressed fracture recover without any means having been employed to raise the bone to its former level, and if he is under seven years of age, the bone will in time be found to have risen of itself and no ill effects will follow injury, but if the person be advanced in life, the bone will not rise and in a few years he will likely to be attacked with epilepsy." "Though depressed fractures will often recover, yet as in the case I have already mentioned, epilepsy may be the consequence subsequently. This it would appear arises from a growth of bone internally, which presses on the brain. I have here a preparation of the skull belonging to this case I alluded to, of the boy who returned to me after several years with epilepsy, and you will see a spicule of bone growing down into the brain. We find these growths of bone into the brain in cases which we cannot trace to any external injury—an exostosis, as it is called, and the subjects of it have, as in the present case, been attacked with epilepsy." This observation of Colles' is now associated with the name of Hughlings Jackson, who described it many decades later. In 1824, Colles published his *Practical precepts on injuries of the head*, which he presented to each of his students. "I have caused to be printed a few practical precepts, of which I beg your acceptance as a mark of my sincere esteem, and a return for your kind attention. The plan of this little book has been borrowed from a similar publication by the late Mr. Dease, the first professor of the practice of surgery in our College. I have ventured to make considerable alterations in the arrangements and much addition to the matter as have been supplied by the present improved state of surgery. I have made Mr. Dease my guide, because every man who has read his larger work, *Observations on wounds of the head*, must see that the principles which he therein inculcates, are now recorded as established truths, and are acted on as rules of practice." The review of Colles' little book in *The Lancet* reads—"Though small and unpretending, it really contains as much useful information as will be generally found in more voluminous treatises on the same subject."

Injuries of the Abdomen. "Suppose you see a portion of protruded bowel with a transverse cut in it—how are you to unite these again? John Bell tells you, you are to put three stitches in it, one at the mesentery, and the other two at equal distance from it and from each other; but when Mr. Bell wrote this it was his imagination rather than his experience which guided him! The fact is, that three stitches in such a wound would be worse than if you had done nothing at all; there would be a drag on these stitches; the mucous membrane would protrude between them and the faeces escape.

When you have the bowels cut either longitudinally or transversely, all you do is to take a small needle and a single thread
and sew the entire wound from end to end with the continued
or glovers suture; you will not have occasion to put card
or candle or anything else into the gut to sew it or keep it
open. Cut the ends of the thread and return the bowels."

Peritonitis. "Do not too readily yield to despair in one of these
cases, for it sometimes happens that after all the surgeon's
hopes have gone, the patient suddenly improves and recovers
completely."

Hernia or Hydocele? "How to distinguish, you are told to
hold a lighted candle on one side of the tumour, and to
throw your eye upon the other; that if the case be water the
tumour will be transparent and you can readily detect it.
This procedure was never recommended by a practical
man"!

Strangulated Hernia. "There are some means by the employment of which you will be able occasionally to relieve a
strangulated hernia without operation, and they should in
most cases be tried before recourse to the knife. You should
begin in these cases by bleeding the patient, not merely
for the purpose of making him feel faint, although this is of
the first importance, but likewise to relieve or moderate inflammation. I never saw a recent strangulated hernia where
bleeding was not necessary. Cases, apparently very similar,
will end differently, so that if your patient, whom you have
bled in the first instance, should afterwards die, you are not
to think that it was the bleeding that killed him. You must
never judge from one or two such cases. My advice to you is,
never let a case of strangulated hernia come across you
without having recourse to bleeding; take blood in a full
stream, and from an orifice so large that you would almost
be afraid to make such a one in a vein. When you make
your patient faint you will often be able to reduce the hernia."
"Tobacco injections are the very best thing after bleeding.
Formerly the smoke of tobacco was used for this purpose,
but the objection to it was the difficulty there often was to
get the machine to work, and the distension it caused was

very disturbing; the infusion is now substituted. You get a drachm of tobacco,* and infuse it for 10–15 minutes in a pint of boiling water; when cool inject one half, and if in a quarter of an hour you observe no effect from it in the system, inject the other; the effect you look for is fainting, depression, cold perspiration, etc. I have seen many cases where the surgeon persevered for a considerable time to try to put up the hernia by the taxis, without success, and where it went up on its own accord after the tobacco enema." "When everything else fails —operate. Do not be misled by other advice, such as waiting for hiccough, peritoneal inflammation, etc. One thing is certain, the result of the French rule of operating within twenty-four hours after its occurrence, is definitely more successful than ours, who wait longer. If operation is necessary the sooner it is done the better." "Sir Charles Bell draws a distinction between strangulation and incarceration, as Bell does not give us any symptoms to enable us to distinguish between strangulation and incarceration to guide our practice; I think he wrote on this subject from observation of one case only!"

On tying a wounded Artery. "You think it would be an easy matter to take it up and tie it! It is not. We may talk as we please about our fine operations, but I protest I do not think in all surgery there is an operation half so difficult as taking up a wounded artery. You have no conception of the difficulties of the case. If you make up your mind that you will not find the artery so superficial as you might from mere anatomical recollections expect, you will get rid of one of the causes of embarrassment; take your time and you will get rid of another."

Popliteal Aneurysm. "Tie the artery where it is about to be crossed by the sartorius muscle. Mr. Hunter, who conceived and established the principle of this operation, tied the artery after it was crossed by the sartorius, but the exact spot does not seem to me to be very clear. The place to tie it, as Scarpa advises, is at the spot where the artery touches the sartorius."

Urethral Stricture. "Stricture is by no means as frequent a

* Shag was preferred to the pigtail variety!

disease as is represented. When I first began to practise in this city, just after Home's book came out, it became quite the fashion in London to have strictures; the fashion soon extended to Dublin and gentlemen in their club-houses had no other conversation but telling each other about their strictures, how often the caustic was applied, etc. Mr. Hunter was of the opinion that caustic might be used for the treatment of strictures, but he limited its use to that part of the urethra anterior to its curve. Sir Everard Home says you may apply it to any part of the canal, but recollect this, that caustic applied according to his plan, will never produce destruction of the texture of the stricture. All that it will, or can do, is merely to cause an increased discharge of mucus, but it never will destroy the substance of a stricture. There is, I am sorry to say, an evident suppression of facts in Sir Everard Home's work. A Frenchman named Ducamp invented a series of instruments for the better application of caustic to strictures. To show you what a pitch of accuracy he aimed at, here is an instrument to measure the *length* of the stricture. Now something like all this might be useful to a pump-borer, but it is not at all adapted to enlighten us on the state of the urethra!''

Hydrocele—the injection method. "First, draw off the fluid. Do not inject—leave. When the hydrocele recurs to a third of its previous size, withdraw the fluid and inject as much port wine and water as was withdrawn. This you suffer to remain until the patient gets faintish, or complains of a kind of uneasiness, not in the testicle, for it is never felt there, but in or about the groin, loins, etc. When this is felt, you let out the wine and the water, or whatever else you injected. Some patients will bear the injection to remain in for a good while, others hardly a moment; but in all cases his sensations must direct you when to let it out. Take care not to withdraw the cannula, or suffer its end to escape from the cavity of the tunica vaginalis, until every drop of the injection comes away, for should any of it get into the scrotum you will be astonished at the terrible effects of inflammation and sloughing that will ensue. After putting the patient to bed, it will sometimes be necessary to give him an anodyne. The first night after the proceeding the patient will not rest as usual. The next day the testicle will be a little swelled and be heavier; sometimes there is a jelly-like softness about the testicle. Keep the patient quiet for ten or twelve days, and ultimately he is perfectly well, as far at least as the hydrocele is considered."

Posterior Curvature of the Spine (Pott's). "A disease which very much resembles psoas abscess, which probably begins in bones and not ligaments. Treat in the horizontal position in bed, for one year or more, country air, proper diet, etc. We are told that it is possible to support the weight of the body from the spine by machinery, and accordingly a great variety of steel apparatus has been contrived. If you pass through the villages of England, you will be astonished at the number of these miserable beings who have been submitted to these machines; as the coach rolls through the town, they all run to the windows to see it, and they really look like wretches in gibbets rather than what they are."

Compound Fractures. "I know nothing in surgery that requires more judgement, more careful discrimination or prompt decision on the part of the surgeon than a case of severe compound fracture. Sometimes the bones themselves will be deadened by the violence, and you will have to amputate on account of this complication, but one piece of advice I give you, never be in a hurry to amputate for a compound fracture, and the experience I have tends to show the ill tendency of early amputation in compound fracture. If you must amputate, wait at least until the symptomatic fever has subsided. Many a very uncompromising case of this kind has turned out without mutilation or other injury, and the operation itself for removing a limb that has sustained a bad compound fracture does not seem to me as successful as might be supposed . . . the man to whom I was a pupil, was very fond of amputation for every kind of compound fracture, and he operated as well as and dexterously as any man I ever knew, yet I never saw a patient in whom he operated on this type of case that did not die in consequence."

Fractures: Non-union. Colles was aware that syphilis, scrofula, pregnancy and cancer were pre-disposing causes of non-union in fractures. "The simplest method of bringing about union, and the one freest from any danger, and which has often been effected, is to try to make the patient walk about a little, using some simple means to keep the upper piece resting perpendicular on the lower . . ."

Fracture of the neck of the Femur. . . . "I have taken pains to investigate this question, and for my own part I must declare I have never found anything like an osseous union of a fracture of the *cervix femoris* . . . . When old people come under your care with this accident, we must treat them very differently from younger ones. When you find that the neck of the femur has been broken more from age than from violence, never tie them up with splints—if you do so, the certain consequence is that they get feverish and restless—they fret— and if you persevere in keeping the splints on, they die in a week. I do not know why this is so, but I have seen it so often. I have had repeated experience of this fact, that there is no doubt in my mind as to the cause and effect. In old people, therefore you should merely, for appearance sake, put a bandage lightly on a limb and support it with pillows— besides, the decided ill effects of splints on aged persons are unnecessary, for in such patients anything like useful union is, of course, not to be thought of."

CHAPTER 8

The Colles Eponyms

.... Ab illo
Dicitur, aeternumque tenet per saecula nomen.*
Virgil.

COLLES' FASCIA

"Now proceed to dissect the perineum. Raise the skin of the perineum, extending the dissection beyond the tuber ischia to the thighs. This exposes to view a strong fascia, which, on dissection, will be found to cover the entire of the perineum, and to blend itself with the structure of the scrotum. This fascia, although on a superficial view it appears continuous with the fascia of the muscles of the thigh, will yet be found, on closer examination, to attach itself very firmly to the rami of the ischium and pubis. The texture and connections of this fascia will serve to explain many of these phenomena attendant on the effusion of urine into the perineum, by rupture or ulceration of the posterior part of the canal of the urethra. First, then, you will find this fluid, when so effused, although it forms a tumour in perineo, rarely terminates by suppuration and ulceration in this spot; being here resisted by the dense and unyielding texture of the fascia, diffusion laterally towards the thighs is prevented by the close attachment of this fascia to the rami of the pubis and ischium; while its progress forwards is favoured by a quantity of cellular substance, interposed between the surface of the perineal muscles and the fascia. In general, then, we find that the urine having caused some tumefaction in perineo, passes on into the scrotum. Here meeting with only a very feeble resistance from the lax texture of this part, it quickly distends it to a very considerable size. In some instances the mischief does not extend further, for suppuration

*It is called after him and preserves his name forever throughout the ages.

takes place in the scrotum, and a quantity of very foetid fluid composed of urine and pus, is discharged as soon as the abscess spontaneously bursts or is opened by the surgeon. In other cases, the effused urine continues its progress until it arrives at the pubis. Here it causes a swelling, which becoming red, tense and painful, at length ulcerates; and giving exit to a large and foetid discharge of urine, mixed with pus, affords some relief to the patient. As often as the patient attempts to pass urine, some of it filters through this opening. In process of time, considerable sloughs of cellular tissue are drawn out through it. After this the swelling subsides, the orifice contracts, and the disease terminates in a urinary fistula . . .''

Abraham Colles—*A Treatise on Surgical Anatomy*, 1811.

John Abernethy (1825) appeared to be unaware of this description when he wrote—"When matter forms in the course of the membranous part of the urethra or in the neighbourhood of the bulb it does not produce inflammation of the skin or break like a common abscess. On the contrary, the skin is but little affected and as the matter increases in quantity it appears kept down as it were collected beneath a fascia . . . . These circumstances indicate that there is a fascia spread beneath the skin of the perineum over the adjacent parts, yet I think the limits of this fascia can scarcely be ascertained by dissection." However, John Struthers (1854) wrote, "The fascia in the perineum is variously called the deep or true superficial fascia, the deep layer of the superficial fascia or the superficial facia. Amongst these various definitions the student is often at a loss to know which structure is being described, and to avoid this source of confusion, and to derive the advantage from the use of a short specific name, I am in the habit of calling it the *Fascia of Colles*, as the general connections of this membrane, and especially the course of infiltrated urine determined by the fascia appear to have been first fully described in this country by the late Abraham Colles of Dublin in his excellent and practical treatise on surgical anatomy."

COLLES' SPACE

The potential space between the perineal membrane above and Colles' Fascia below, containing the crura of the penis, the bulb of urethra, and their attendant muscles, the scrotal vessels and nerves and the superficial transversus perinei muscle is referred to as the Colles' Space (McNalty).

THE COLLES LIGAMENT OF INGUINAL HERNIA

"The wall of the abdomen immediately behind this (external abdominal) ring consists of the conjoined tendons of the transversalis and internal oblique muscles and of the transversalis fascia, the natural strength of which at this spot is increased by their attachment to the crest of the pubis, and by the connection which the outer edge of the rectus has with the fascia transversalis. An additional security is derived from two small but strong fasciae, between which the cord passes; one of these is the fascia, so often mentioned, which stretching from one pillar of the ring to the other fills up all that part of it which is above the spermatic cord. The other is a strong triangular fascia, arising by a pretty broad base, from the crest of the pubis, anteriorly to the insertion of the internal oblique and transversalis tendons, passing immediately behind the external abdominal muscle until it reaches the linea alba, in which it terminates by a narrow point about one and a half inches above the pubis. The edge of this fascia, which looks towards the spermatic cord, is slightly grooved, or hollowed out. When the abdominal muscles and the linea alba are stretched, this ridge of the ligament is seen to rise up from the pubis and consequently to shut up a greater portion of the external ring. Another advantage derived from this ligament is that it strengthens the insertion of the tendons of the internal oblique and transversalis into the pubis."

Then with characteristic honesty Colles continues:

"This fascia is delineated but not marked in plate first of Mr. Astley Cooper's treatise on inguinal hernia, nor is it noticed in his descriptions."

Abraham Colles—*A Treatise on Surgical Anatomy*, 1811.

McCoy (1845) referred to this structure as *The Colles Ligament of Inguinal Hernia*, a description still used in Dublin. Harrison

(1848) and Macalister (1884) named it the *Triangular Ligament (or Fascia) of Colles*. In modern anatomical nomenclature it is known simply as the "reflected part of the inguinal ligament".

THE COLLES FASCIA OF FEMORAL HERNIA

"At the point (where the saphena dips deep to gain the femoral vein) we observe that the fascia lata, which in all the lower part of the limb had formed one general covering or sheath for the muscles of the thigh, divides into two parts. One of these closely invests the muscles which arise from the pubes, while the other covers those which lie on the iliac or outer side of the limb. The former we call the pubic or pectineal portion; the latter, the outer or iliac portion of the fascia lata . . . . The outer part of the fascia lata covering the muscles on the external or iliac side of the limb, lies above the plane of the pubic portion, especially in the vicinity of the femoral vessels; for here the iliac portion will be found to pass before, while the pubic portion passes behind them . . . Of the pubic portion, we shall merely say that it is more thin than the external part, that it is attached superiorly to the anterior edge of the pubis above the origin of the pectineus muscle, that it gives a close covering to the muscles which arise from the pubis. The external portion demands more of our attention, for it will be found so intimately connected with crural hernia as to have a material influence on the symptoms and treatment of the disease. That part of the iliac portion of the fascia lata which runs between the femoral vein and the symphysis of the pubis, has its upper edge blended with Poupart's ligament, from which it descends to the pubic fascia; it is seen to turn upwards under Poupart's ligament, so as to touch the fascia at a point nearer to the crest of the pubis than the line of Poupart's ligament. The iliac and pubic fascia united, then continue their course upwards until they insert themselves into the crest of the pubis."

Abraham Colles—*A Treatise on Surgical Anatomy*, 1811.

It is this extension of the iliac part of the fascia lata, named by Croly (1895) *The Colles Fascia of Femoral Hernia*, applied to the medial wall of the femoral sheath, that Colles demonstrated to be the constricting agent in strangulated femoral hernia, and not the crescentric margin of Gimbernat's ligament which lies above and medial to the femoral ring, and therefore taking no part in the constriction. The *Colles' Operation* for strangulated femoral hernia is division of this fascia on the medial side; it is the operation we perform in practice today, although regrettably many surgeons erroneously believe that they are carrying out the Gimbernat operation.

COLLES' FRACTURE

On the Fracture of the carpal extremity of the radius.

"The injury to which I wish to direct the attention of surgeons, has not, as far as I know, been described by any author; indeed, the form of the carpal extremity of the radius would rather incline us to question its being liable to fracture. The absence of crepitus, and of other common symptoms of fracture, together with the swelling which instantly arises in this, as in other injuries of the wrist, render the difficulty of ascertaining the real nature of the case very considerable. This fracture takes place at about an inch and a half above the carpal extremity of the radius, and exhibits the following appearances. The posterior surface of the limb presents a considerable deformity; for a depression is seen in the forearm, about an inch and a half above the end of this bone, while a considerable swelling occupies the wrist and the metacarpus. Indeed, the carpus and base of metacarpus appear to be thrown backward so much, as on first view to excite a suspicion that the carpus has been dislocated forward.

"On viewing the anterior surface of the limb, we observe a considerable fullness, as if caused by the flexor tendons being thrown forwards. The fullness extends upwards to about one third of the length of the forearm, and terminates below at the upper edge of the annular ligament of the wrist. The extremity of the ulna is seen projecting towards the palm and inner edge of the limb; the degree, however, in which this projection takes place, is different in different instances.

"If the surgeon proceed to investigate the nature of this injury, he will find that the end of the ulna admits of being readily moved backwards and forwards. On the posterior surface, he will discover, by the touch, that the swelling on the wrist and metacarpus is not caused entirely by an effusion among the softer parts; he will perceive that the ends of the metacarpal, and second row of carpal bones, form no small part of it. This, strengthening the suspicion which the first view of the case had excited, leads him to examine, in a more particular manner, the anterior part of the joint; but the want of that solid resistance, which a dislocation of the carpus forward must occasion, forces him to abandon this notion, and leaves him in a state of perplexing uncertainty as to the real nature of the injury. He will therefore endeavour to gain some information, by examining the bones of the forearm. The facility with which (as was before noticed) the ulna can be moved backward and forward, does not furnish him with any useful hint. When he moves his fingers along the anterior surface of the radius, he finds it more full and prominent than is natural; a similar examination of the posterior surface of this bone, induces him to think that a depression is felt about an inch and a half above its carpal extremity. He now expects to find satisfactory proofs of a fracture of the radius at this spot. For this purpose, he attempts to move the broken pieces of the bone in opposite directions; but, although the patient is by this examination subjected to considerable pain, yet, neither crepitus nor a yielding of the bone at the seat of fracture, nor any other positive evidence of the existence of such an injury is thereby obtained. The patient complains of severe pain as often as an attempt is made to give to the limb the motions of pronation and supination.

"If the surgeon lock his hand in that of the patient's, and make extension, even with a moderate force, he restores the limb to its natural form, but the distortion of the limb instantly returns on the extension being removed. Should the facility with which a moderate extension restores the limb to its form, induce the practitioner to treat this as a case of sprain, he will find, after a lapse of time sufficient for the removal of similar swellings, the deformity undiminished. Or, should he mistake the case for a dislocation of the wrist, and attempt to retain the parts *in situ* by tight bandages and splints, the pain caused by the pressure on the back of the wrist will force him to unbind them in a few hours; and, if they be applied more loosely, he will find, at the expiration of a few weeks, that the deformity still exists in its fullest extent, and that it is now no longer to be removed by making extension of the limb. By such mistakes the patient is doomed to endure for many months considerable lameness and stiffness of the limb, accompanied by severe pains on attempting to bend the hand and fingers. One consolation only remains, that the limb will at some remote period again enjoy perfect freedom in all its motions and be completely exempt from pain; the deformity, however, will remain undiminished through life.

"The unfavourable result of some of the first cases of this description which came under my care, forced me to investigate with peculiar anxiety the nature of the injury. But while the absence of crepitus and of the other usual symptoms of fracture rendered the diagnosis extremely difficult, a recollection of the superior strength and thickness of this part of the radius, joined to the mobility of its articulation with the carpus and ulna, rather inclined me to question the possibility of a fracture taking place at this part of the bone. At last, after many unsuccessful trials, I hit upon the following simple method of examination, by which I was enabled to ascertain, that the symptoms above enumerated actually arose from a fracture, seated about an inch and a half above the carpal extremity of the radius. Let the surgeon apply the fingers of one hand to the seat of the suspected fracture, and, locking the other hand in that of the patient, make a moderate extension, until he observes the limb restored to its natural form. As soon as this is effected, let him move the patient's hand backward and forward; and he will, at every such attempt, be sensible of a yielding of the fractured ends of of the bone, and this to such a degree as must remove all doubt from his mind.

"The nature of this injury once ascertained, it will be a very easy matter to explain the different phenomena attendant on it, and to point out a method of treatment which will prove completely successful. The hard swelling which appears on the back of the hand, is caused by the carpal surface of the radius being directed slightly backwards instead of looking directly downwards. The carpus and metacarpus, retaining their connections with this bone, must follow it in its derangements, and cause the convexity above alluded to. This change of direction in the articulating surface of the radius is caused by the tendons of the extensor muscles of the thumb, which pass along the posterior surface of the radius in sheaths firmly connected with the inferior extremity of this bone. The broken extremity of the radius being thus drawn backwards, causes the ulna to appear prominent towards the palmar surface, while it is possibly thrown more towards the inner or ulnar side of the limb, by the upper end of the fragment of the radius pressing against it in that direction. The separation of these two bones from each other is facilitated by a previous rupture of their capsular ligament; an event which may readily be occasioned by the violence of the injury. An effusion into the sheaths of the flexor tendons will account for that swelling which occupies the limb anteriorly.

"It is obvious that, in the treatment of this fracture, our attention should be principally directed to guard against the carpal end of the radius being drawn backwards. For this purpose, while assistants hold the limb in a middle state between pronation and supination, let a thick and firm compress be applied transversely on the anterior surface of the limb, at the seat of fracture, taking care that it shall not press on the ulna; let this be bound on firmly with a roller, and then let a tin splint, formed to the shape of the arm, be applied to both its anterior and posterior surfaces. In cases where the end of the ulna has appeared much displaced, I have laid a very narrow wooden splint along the naked side of this bone. This latter splint, I now think, should be used in every instance, as, by pressing the extremity of the ulna against the side of the radius, it will tend to oppose the displacement of the fractured end of this bone. It is scarcely necessary to observe, that the two principal splints should be much more narrow at the wrist than those in general use, and should also extend to the roots of the fingers, spreading out so as to give a firm support to the hand. The cases treated on this plan have all recovered without the smallest defect or deformity of the limb, in the ordinary time for the cure of fractures.

"I cannot conclude these observations without remarking, that were my opinion to be drawn from these cases only which have occurred to me, I should consider this as by far the most common injury to which the wrist or carpal extremities of the radius and ulna are exposed. During the last three years I have not met with a single instance of Desault's dislocation of the inferior end of the radius, while I have had the opportunities of seeing a vast number of the fracture of the lower end of this bone."

Abraham Colles—*Edinb. med. and surg. J.* (1814): *10*: 182.

This famous classical paper was rescued from oblivion by Robert William Smith (1847) in his *Treatise on Fractures in the Vicinity of Joints*—"It is certainly very extraordinary that although the pathology and treatment of this injury were fully and accurately described by Mr. Colles so long back as April, 1814, not a single British or foreign author who has written since has made the slightest reference to Mr. Colles' name in connection with the subject, even when almost quoting his words." Smith was naturally saddened by the omission of any reference to Colles' paper in the writings of Astley Cooper, who describing the fracture wrote—"The lower fragment of the radius is seen in its natural position attached to the carpus and hand, while the lower end of the upper fragment is displaced forward into the flexor tendons", and continues "I have seen the accident frequently and at first did not exactly understand the nature of the injury; indeed dissection alone taught me its real character!" Cooper's misinterpretations of the displacement of the fragments were even illustrated by a drawing of a specimen from the museum of St. Thomas' Hospital, and were perpetuated in the writings of his adulatory nephew, Bransby Cooper, who actually incurred such a fracture of his own wrist.

Smith corrected some minor errors in Colles' description of the fracture. The fracture line was placed too high, it was in the weakest and not in the strongest part of the bone, and finally the carpal surface of the radius not only looks downwards but also forwards and inwards. Incidentally, Smith supported the non-impaction theory of this fracture, which was later to be corrected by his successor, Edward Hallaran Bennett (of the metacarpal fracture) who demonstrated no less than fifty-six specimens of Colles' fracture at a B.M.A. meeting in Cork in 1879. Smith in his book describes and illustrates the "reversed" Colles' fracture, now known as Smith's fracture, resulting from force applied to the back of the wrist.

En passant, we should salute Robert William Smith, one of the most distinguished anatomists and surgeons of his generation. A Trinity graduate, and a licentiate of the Surgeons' School, he was a student of and later surgeon to the Richmond Hospital, Dublin, and in 1849 was appointed the first professor of surgery in Trinity. He was an original investigator of the first order and his numerous contributions to surgical literature were of the highest quality. The principal founder of the Pathological Society of Dublin—the oldest society of its kind in the British Isles (and now continued as the Pathology Section of the Royal Academy of Medicine in Ireland)—Smith was its secretary until his death in 1873. An eloquent speaker at medical gatherings, a brilliant linguist, so enthusiastic was he as a teacher that he latterly almost completely abandoned practice so that he might devote more time to study and to the instruction of his classes. His success in the chair of surgery decided Trinity in 1858 to institute degrees in that subject—the first University in these islands to do so, and against the opposition of the Royal Colleges. Smith was Vice-President of the Surgeons' College when he died. We will also remember him as the man who carried out the post mortem examination on his old friend and teacher, Abraham Colles.

COLLES' LAW

"The following facts appears to me very deserving of notice— I have never seen or heard of a single instance in which a syphilitic infant, (although its mouth be ulcerated) suckled by his own mother, had produced ulceration of her breasts; whereas very few instances have occurred where a syphilitic infant had not infected a strange hired wet nurse, and who had been previously in good health. It is a curious fact, that I never witnessed nor ever heard of an instance in which a child deriving the infection of syphilis from its parents has caused an ulceration of the breast of its mother."

Abraham Colles—*Practical observations on the venereal disease and on the use of mercury.* London (1837).

It was Diday (1869) who first used the term "Colles' law", referring to its author as "the most enlightened, most modest and learned", and continued, "but I repeat, it would be necessary to ransack very diligently the annals of science to discover a fact equivalent to this one. We are, therefore, fully justified in asserting that a child born syphilitic through the agency of its parents never communicates the disease to his mother who suckles it." Hutchinson (1887) referred to Colles' law as a remarkable observation, and continues—"since Colles' day no exceptions to this law have, I think, been put on record which are worthy of trust". Diday, Hutchinson and even Colles himself gave examples of cases which were exceptions to this law, and of course we now know that the law is fallacious and of historical interest only. Although this law was original the observation on which it was founded had been made many years earlier. Still, in his *History of Pediatrics* (London, 1931) gives the following quotation from a treatise on the care of children by Simon de Vallambert, published in 1565.

"I saw at Tours a goldsmith who for 14 or 15 years since he had the Great Pox had felt no ill at all and seemed quite well, nevertheless all his children that he has had since then had the Pox soon after they were born, at seven or eight days old, and gave it to their nurse although the mother was an honest woman well spoken of, who strangely enough had never taken the disease from her husband and had not been affected in any way."

COLLES' PUSTULES

In a series of fatal cases resulting in wounds received in dissection, Colles in describing the skin changes remarks— "Another remarkable feature was the very peculiar appearance of the pustules (unlike to any I had ever witnessed) and the striking resemblance of the pustules to one another. Add to this the appearance of a similar pustule on the forearm of Mr. Dease (Colles' co-professor, who was one of the victims). The character of this pustule could not have been influenced by the wound of the lancet, for that wound had only the ordinary appearance observed in cases where a slight inflammation supervened on bloodletting; besides, this pustule was seated lower down on the limb, and the skin intervening between it and the wound remained perfectly natural, free from discolouration, swelling or pain. The elevations of the cuticle to the eye resembling vesications, while actually solid, and the swelling of the forearm, which was opened only a few hours before death, present characters which tend still further to remove the resemblance of this to any other disease usually consequent upon wounds."

Abraham Colles—*Dubl. Hosp. Reports* (1822): *3*: 203.

Graves (1848) referred to these as "Colles' Pustules"— "Vesicles and pustules similar to those produced in dissection wounds, and other diseases produced by the introduction of animal poison into the system, may arise from the action of morbid changes spontaneously occurring in the body, is a fact which admits of being proved, and opens to us a new and interesting field of enquiry. Thus, in the case of typhus, where the effect of pressure or some other accident has occasioned bedsores of a bad character, and even where no bedsores are present, I have on several occasions seen low secondary fever produced and have observed vesicles or pustules appear on the skin similar to those described by Mr. Colles as accompanying the fever of dissection wounds."

COLLES' CINNEBAR CANDLES

"Cinnebar or grey oxide of mercury is to be mixed with melted wax and with a cotton wick be moulded into a small candle. This may be stuck on a common plate and then burnt under a curved glass funnel, which is to be raised about an inch from the plate. By conducting the process in this way, we are certain that all the mercury is consumed, which is but seldom effected in the ordinary mode of throwing it on heated metal; the fumes, too, are thus more gradually brought in contact with the diseased surfaces, and the patient, if fatigued, may blow out the candle and suspend the process until he feels able to resume it."

Abraham Colles—*Practical observations on the venereal disease and on the use of mercury.* London (1837).

COLLES' "COPPER" RETRACTORS

These malleable spatulas of prince's metal were first introduced by Colles in his operation of tying the subclavian artery (1815). Robert Liston (1820) wrote—"I consider them as the greatest addition made to our surgical instruments for many years".

CHAPTER 9

Colles the Man

"It is the personal alone, Sir, that interests mankind."

Dr. Johnson.

Careers of the greatest usefulness are often those which present fewest of those striking incidents and uncommon situations, which most readers covet in a personal memoir; and it is pre-eminently the nature of the medical profession to withdraw its practitioners from the conspicuous places of life. In no other callings are the exhibition of skill and evidence of genius so far removed from the public view. In no other profession are the steps by which celebrity is attained so secret, or is it so difficult to construct an interesting narrative out of details of intellectual exertion, though crowned with the most eminent success. Medical biography accordingly forms a very interesting portion of that branch of literature which records the lives and preserves the intellectual portraits of distinguished medical men. Even a rapid and imperfect sketch of one who, while living, was the object in a high degree of their respect and admiration, cannot fail to be interesting to the members of his own profession. To young men about to start in the same arduous course, an outline of a career so honourable is peculiarly instructive. Colles won his way to eminence by means which are, to some extent, within the reach of all. He may be said to have wrested success from the hands of adverse fortune by his energy and indomitable perseverance.

Colles would scarcely have remembered his father, who died before he was six years old. His mother was a remarkable woman. Left with three young sons, and a daughter, she kept the family marble business going and determined to give her children the very best education then available in the country. She endowed her children with Christian principles, with the

love of home and family life, and presided over that extraordinary united family for a further sixty years, dying in 1840
at the age of ninety. Abraham, or in family circles "Aby",
was probably her favourite son, no doubt due to his childhood
illnesses and his long periods away from home. Some very
affectionate letters passed between them, especially from
Edinburgh. She gave him a full account of her own illnesses,
seeking advice for her fainting attacks, her biliousness, her
bowels; and on one occasion was to receive the reply, "As to
your question *What am I to do for the itch?* I must tell you that
the practice here which seems to be most pleasant to the
generality of patients in that distemper is to *scratch*!" In later
years there was a continuous stream of prescriptions and
medicines passing between St. Stephen's Green and Millmount,
and when Abraham himself could not get down to see her at
Kilkenny, he advised that in case of any new symptoms she
was at once to consult young Alcock, the local practitioner—
"an intelligent and active young man, one whom I have known
to have studied his profession very diligently and with the most
ample opportunities". Incidentally, this Benjamin Alcock
(of the canal) was a Kilkenny man and had been Colles'
apprentice and brilliant pupil. He was later to become the first
professor of anatomy at the new Queen's College, Cork, in
1849, but eventually emigrated to the United States.

It was but natural that Abraham looked up to his elder
brother William for guidance in his career. William was regarded as the "intellectual" of the family. Brilliant in Trinity,
as a prizeman and scholar of the house, and in the debates of
the College Historical Society, he finally clashed with the
establishment and left without a degree. He would now be
classed as a left wing intellectual backing many causes that
called out for reform, but was never militant. With leanings
towards law and local politics, he never took either seriously
enough to emerge as a leader, preferring to remain in the
background to advise the leaders on such great issues as the
payment of tithes, and Catholic emancipation, and lived to see
his principles triumphant. He was on terms of close friendship
with Daniel O'Connell—the "Liberator"—and had similar
political views on the repeal of the Union, as this letter shows:

"My Dear Colles,

You see I have taken, or endeavoured to take, your hint. I did as well as I could, and according to my policy I will repeat the idea in many forms before I think I have fully complied with your suggestion. Sensitive men—and most men of talent are so—shrink from the repetition of the same thought. As far as the public are concerned, it is a great mistake. It is necessary to say the same thing one hundred times before the public *catch it*. But then it becomes identified with the public mind—so I delude myself.

For Heaven's sake why do you not attend a meeting of the Citizen's Club, and give us the benefit of one sarcastic, argumentative, interesting speech against the Union? Do not answer the question, but think of it.

Very faithfully yours,

21st August, 1840.   Daniel O'Connell."

Abraham consulted William for advice and guidance when he was applying for the College chairs.

"Stewart and McEvoy asked me, did I mean to propose myself in the next election for the College chairs? I told them *I thought not*. McEvoy said he thought it a duty that every member who was qualified for office owed to the College. On my objecting to the large family that Halahan had and the length of time he held the place, and on account of the injury it must do to Dease and Halahan to be removed from such a situation, McEvoy replied that he felt and thought that I should state it so to the electors and leave it to them whether they will be guided by these considerations. Since then I have spoken to Obré. He can see no difficulty and no impropriety in it, he thinks that every man should exert his talents on his own behalf and cannot see why I should make any objection to offering myself as a candiate. I have seen Stewart. He says that he is agitated between public good and a private feeling for those other men (the present professors). He wishes that we could make it a triplet and talks of my giving Halahan a sum of money annually in lieu of his part of the profits. He wishes to have some conversation with

McEvoy on the subject, but seems determined on bringing me in, if possible with the consent of the present professors, if not against their consent. I wish to know whether you see any impropriety in my offering myself for the office. I sometimes think that I am over delicate in the matter, at other times I fear that a sense of present interest prevents my seeing anything which may be unfair in my making such an attempt. Write soon and give me your opinion.

P.S. Tell Rachel that my horse has not since shown any sign of lameness."

In a subsequent letter to William (August, 1804) Abraham wrote: "The time is fast approaching which is to decide on the fate and fame of your brother the doctor. Yesterday Mr. Halahan's letter of resignation was read to the court and passed off with very few remarks. On Saturday or Monday I hope that my proposal will be read. I submit the following for your correction and request an answer by the earliest opportunity. I know you will exert yourself, as you can readily conceive the great mental anxiety which must attend the merest trifles in matters of such consequence."

"To the Court of Censors, etc. ———

Gentlemen,

Having learned that Mr. Halahan declines offering himself on the ensuing election as a candidate for one of the professorships of anatomy and surgery in your College, I beg leave to submit myself to your consideration in his room. As the arrangement laid down in the printed syllabus already approved of by you seems to be unexceptional, I have not thought it necessary to trouble you with any other on the present occasion. Should my proposal fortunately be honoured by your approbation, be assured, Gentlemen, that I shall labour by the most unremitting assiduity in discharging the duties of this office to justify your choice and to manifest my gratitude.

I have the honour to be, etc.

A.C."

"P.S. Let me have your answer as soon as possible. Will you let me know if the lime water has cured my mother's mare. I am interested not a little in the answer, as I yesterday bought a broken-winded mare which was going off a great bargain. My friend Merrick bought her for me. I hope she will answer me very well for this winter, and therefore I wish that Dick would sell Bardolph in the most beneficial time and manner that he can, or if he and you think him worth keeping until next spring for my own use—let him remain on Dick's grass a little longer. Tell Rachel of the change in my plan of jockeyship and let her immediately acquaint Tom with it."

In 1806 Abraham asked William for his opinion on his introductory lectures—later to be published in his surgical anatomy.

"To offer my apologies for sending you such *a barbarous jargon* and such unconnected ideas, would not evince the strong reliance I have in your wishes to promote my success in life. Be assured that neither indolence nor dissipation have prevented it from being much better. Will you let me know of the plan, etc., provided that you can give *a critical analysis of chaos*. I need not say that you cannot too speedily or too strongly turn the whole body of your thoughts into this channel. My mind cannot be easy until I feel myself in possession of my twelve introductory lectures.

P.S. Tell Dick that I wish he would take that vicious little mare from me and cure her. Let him give whatever he thinks she is worth. I wish that he could send for her soon as she eats hay with a good appetite. My friend, Mr. Bowers, will be in Kilkenny in a few days and will take down to you a silver watch, which I hope you will wear in preference to that which you now have. I can only offer two inducements, one is that it will chance to tell the hour occasionally, which yours never has done, and another is that you will oblige me by wearing it. As this is the first present I have ventured to offer to you, I hope that you will treat it with more than your usual kindness to presents."

In 1809, Abraham wrote to William—

"I intend to publish a set of plates designed to show the relative position of the principal arteries of the body, and the nature and depths of the parts to be cut through by the surgeon in his attempts to tie a ligature on them. These plates, of course will be accompanied by explanations, and I may be led to offer some practical remarks of mine own— these, however will be but few. By this hasty outline you may perceive that the principal labour devolves on my painter and engraver—that the only merit I can assume, is from being the first to supply a deficiency which yet exists in anatomical plates, and from doing this in such a way as will at once display the artery and point out its relative position and the parts interposed between it and the surface. The advantages which I may reap cannot lie in the sale of the book, for altho' I expect that very many copies will be sold, yet engravings are so dear as always to leave the publisher at some loss. The profession may be benefited—the students by having these plates to assist them in the dissecting room, and the practitioner by having it in his power, at a single glance, to refresh his anatomical knowledge and prepare for operations which are now considered as the most critical and alarming. The only person to whom I have disclosed my design is Comeford, the painter, and him I have bound up to strict secrecy. Do not communicate my intentions to *any* person—for you see that once the plan is known it would be an easy matter to anticipate me. You see, then, that like some ladies who have held themselves too high, I am obliged after some years to come down and be satisfied with the credit of having published a useful rather than an astonishing work."

It is unlikely that Colles carried out his plan, as no specimens of these drawings or engravings now appear to exist.

The correspondence between Abraham and his brother William was not always one-sided. William had a little business of manufacturing notepaper from linen rags and it was Abraham who was constantly advising him on its management, and was ever sending him specimens, information, and quotations of the rival manufacturers in Dublin. Abraham also acted as

William's medical adviser. "I am sorry to find that you have again been visited by your earthly torments. Peggy Bates, relying on the plenitudes of my medical powers, desires me to send all the necessary directions for the treatment of your complaint, but you know too well how slender are my means. I think, however, you should bathe your feet every night for four or five successive nights, in horse-radish water and take morning and mid-day a tablespoonful of tincture of senna in two spoonsful of water. This, together with a tolerably large dose of patience, is all I can recommend!" On another occasion he advised William to have blood taken "in a full stream". William, however, did not take life seriously, although on one occasion he did fight a duel. He remained an Irish country gentleman, collecting his rents, friendly with everyone in the Kilkenny district, and passed his life with ease. He died a bachelor in 1849.

Abraham was equally attached to his younger brother, Richard (of Riverview, later known as Laristown House, County Kilkenny). When Richard completed his education at Kilkenny College he went to live with his uncle in Dublin with a view to entering on a commercial career there; but after a short time he, about the year 1795, decided to return home to Kilkenny in order to take up and carry on the marble business, which his mother, with partial success, kept going from the time of his father's death; a decision from which she (apparently having no strong faith in its future) in vain tried to dissuade him. His character being, like that of his brother Abraham, a resolute one, and his mind being fully made up on this subject, all her arguments against his intention proved to be futile. Fortunately, he was justified by the result. Napoleon's blockade of British commerce gave Richard his opportunity, as it had the effect of keeping foreign marble out of Britain. He had consequently a demand for Kilkenny marble, at a very lucrative price, and in as great quantities as he could supply. There are many records of the efficiency of the business and the excellence of its products. Away in Scotland (1795–1797) Abraham was often seeking contacts and contracts for his brother's business from Edinburgh and Glasgow firms. The marble business, however, was not so prosperous after the Napoleonic war, with the re-entry of foreign marble into Britain, and in Ireland there was famine, fever, and political unrest, which made things difficult for many years afterwards. Richard married Anne Harper in 1810—the year he built Riverview House. He had a family of four sons and seven daughters, and died in 1849 within a few days of his brother William. His lineal descendants today are Capt. A. C. Colles, R.N., and Commander Sir Dudley Colles, K.C.B., K.C.V.O., R.N., Extra Equerry to H.M.

Rachel, naturally, was her mother's darling and adored by her brothers. She married the Reverend Thomas Ottiwell Moore, D.D. rector of Liskenfere, County Wexford, in 1804, and there were eleven children of the marriage. One of their descendants was the late Thomas Ottiwell Graham, a respected leader of the surgical profession in Dublin and president of his College 1942–44.

The most important event in the family scene was the marriage of Abraham to Sophia, daughter of the Reverend Jonathan Cope, Rector of Ahascragh, County Galway, on the 27th April, 1807. Abraham was then thirty-four years old, and Sophia was twenty-five. By all accounts she was a charming, educated, cultured daughter of the rectory, and for Abraham his one and only love. His letters to her have survived and one cannot read these without emotion. To him she was, for their thirty-six years together, ever "my dearest girl". Even short separations caused him intense anxiety for her welfare, and he was unable to concentrate on his work until her return. For Abraham, family and home was everything, and Sophia was a perfect wife and mother. He died in her arms. They had eleven children, one daughter dying in infancy and one son in teenage, but all other nine children reached adult state (see Appendix). The present "head of the family" is Ronald M. Colles, the lineal descendant of Henry, the second son of Abraham Colles.

Sometime after marriage, Sophia was recuperating in Millmount, probably from a miscarriage, and Abraham, ever conscious of her absence, sent this reminder to his bachelor brother William.

"I know that you will readily excuse one of my uxorious disposition if I presume to give you a hint for your conduct towards her—it is that you refrain from any strong allusion or pointed insinuation to love affairs. She is a woman of much delicacy and though she did not speak of you and Dick, yet I am sure that she must have been annoyed by some things of this nature when you were last in town, because I have heard censure of others who were not so pointed in their conversations. You may possibly think me strangely altered, but I do not know that I am. Surely you and Dick would not do anything which would render my woman's time less pleasant at Millmount. From what has lately happened, she will be more than usually delicate on such points. Tell Dick that he will oblige me by driving her out in the gig as often as he conveniently can, and in return I will walk his wife over all the beauties of Dublin. Sophia must not go to many of the plays, as her recovery will be retarded and my annoyance continued. For more reasons than one I cannot go to see any of the plays this winter."

The steady growth of Colles' practice is well shown by his fee book, which Kirkpatrick must have seen. In the year of his marriage his total fees amounted to £754 16s. 3½d. In the following year they were £1,160 9s. 4d.; in 1811 they were over £2,000; in 1814 over £3,000; in 1820 over £4,000; in 1823 over £5,000, and in 1826 they amounted to £6,168 9s. 7½d. In the forty-six years of his practice his fees from patients amounted to £151,191 3s. 3d. As his individual fees were as a rule small, and as much of his time was necessarily devoted to his duties as professor at the Surgeons' School and as surgeon to Dr. Steevens' Hospital, we can well believe that Colles was an indefatigable worker.

For some five years before his marriage Abraham lived at No. 71 Dame Street. He and Sophia were now to set up home at No. 11 St. Stephen's Green. Later, as his practice and family increased, they moved to a larger house, No. 21 St. Stephen's Green, which became their permanent home. This lovely Georgian house was later occupied by his sons, William and Henry; then it became St. Andrews College, and later still the government Estate Office. Recently, it has suffered the same fate as much of Georgian Dublin by being demolished and rebuilt as offices. With his large family he found it necessary to purchase a "country" residence in Donnybrook, then a small village outside Dublin. This "Donnybrook Cottage" had large grounds, and there in the midst of servants, nannies, horses, ponies, governesses, gardeners, grooms and gigs, his children enjoyed a happy upbringing, especially in the summer time. In an age when men invested their money in land, Colles bought many small farms in Kilkenny and neighbouring counties, and eight of his County Carlow properties alone brought him a yearly rental of £329 12d. 6d. He acquired also one large estate, Bonnettstown Hall, Kilkenny, for £2,000, although he never appears to have resided there. In all these transactions his brothers were his advisers and rent collectors. Abraham also had a share in the family property and business, but there was never the slightest friction between the brothers, and Abraham often lent them large sums of money for their various enterprises.

In his younger days Colles rode to Kilkenny on horseback in thirty-six hours, usually breaking the journey at Newbridge. The stage coach at that time was very overcrowded, requiring six horses and running hours late, and for travelling between the two cities Colles arranged his horse transport privately between members of the family and their friends. In Dublin his horse carriage was well known, but it was without the ornate trappings of Kirby's famous coach. Colles rarely visited Britain and there are only two records of journeys to London and Glasgow on College business.

As his professional status grew his services were much in demand, and there were many records of him travelling long and late to far distant counties to see patients, especially medical practitioners and their friends. For many years he was the favourite surgeon for consultation, particularly for his juniors, and there were many hundreds of these throughout Ireland. He owed this honourable preference to their profound conviction that, while they availed themselves of his experience, their characters and interests were safe in his hands. During a practice of duration and extent not often equalled, he was never known to make a remark or as much as throw out a hint, in consultation, tending to prejudice the reputation or hurt the feelings of the most inexperienced practitioner who sought his aid. With such intellectual and moral qualifications his advance was naturally rapid. The principal features of his character were little calculated to catch the public eye or to attract idle curiosity. He was an accomplished gentleman in the truest sense of the word, amiable, upright, modest, intellectual, seemingly unconscious of the high estimation in which he was held by those around him; simple in manners, cheerful in disposition, of the most kindly good nature, endowed with the charm of natural courtesy which made him the delight of his friends and absolutely the idol of his own family circle. An acute observer, eminently sagacious, he knew the world well, but was not corrupted by it. Having a healthy and well-balanced mind, he possessed solid judgment, sound understanding, and the kindest of hearts. He was a man of rare benevolence, a generous giver, ever forestalling solicitation, and sparing the pain of an appeal. His contemporaries tell us that he was above middle size, his figure well proportioned, and his manner unaffectedly dignified. He had a shrewd, clear, good eye, a fine forehead, and a character of marked decision around the mouth. He was an early riser from the beginning of his career. He liked rural retirement, and preferred the society of his own house and intercourse with his intimate friends to all other pleasures.

From 1799 when he was elected a member of the Royal College of Surgeons, until his retirement from the College chair of surgery in 1836, Colles took an active part in the affairs of his College and lived to see it enjoy a European reputation. Much of its celebrity was unquestionably due to the energy with which Colles devoted himself to its improvements. He attended its meetings with scrupulous regularity, and was always ready to relinquish lucrative employment when his presence at its council was required. The affection which he bore that institution was almost parental, and it is not too much to say that it was returned with filial veneration. It is obvious, likewise, that the man who did so much to reform and extend the system of surgical instruction had large claims upon public gratitude. Colles never ceased to impress upon his contemporaries that the greatest object of those who founded the College, as well as the purpose of the legislature which chartered and endowed it, was to advance the science of surgery, increase the respectability of the profession by raising the standards of previous require- ments, and, above all, secure to the public the constant supply of practitioners as highly educated as possible, familiar with every modern improvement or discovery, trained under expert masters, instructed by the ablest lecturers and tried by the test of the most rigorous examinations. In his attachment to the College of Surgeons, there was no narrow *esprit de corps;* still less was he influenced by any regard for his personal importance. He considered the College an instrument for the attainment of high objects, and laboured strenuously to make that instrument as brilliant and effective as possible. Many valuable forms and improvements, especially the establishment of new chairs in chemistry, botany and medical jurisprudence, were the result of his zeal, activity and foresight. The best rules and constitu- tions were the offspring of his prudence and sagacity, and there is scarcely an instance of his advice having been rejected, or of any plan which he recommended having failed to carry the suffrages of the great majority of that body.

No man less than Colles took a tradesman's view of his profession. He nevertheless always spoke of it to his pupils as a calling wherein honourable men, striving to gain a livelihood, confer advantages upon themselves by their service to the public. We frequently find passages similar to the follow- ing in the manuscript notes of his lectures:

"Let the history of this establishment (the College of Sur- geons) serve to animate your exertions. See what progress the science and practice of surgery have made within the few years since the foundation of this institution; progress which must in justice be ascribed to the enthusiastic zeal, pro- found good sense, and incorruptible integrity of a few indivi- duals. See how these men, by promoting the progress of science, have at the same time raised the profession and its members to a rank in society far beyond what even their fondest wishes could have anticipated. Be assured that in this, more than in any other walk of life, public benefit and private advantage are so blended together that the most certain means of advancing your private interest is to promote the public good. Be assured, by manly fortitude and determined perseverance, you will sooner or later overcome every obstacle, and thus render your future career of practice not only lucrative but honourable to yourselves and most useful to the community."

His character as a lecturer was high; yet it is not easy to state with precision in what his excellence consisted. As a young student he applied himself to the art of public speaking in the College Historical Society of Trinity, and later in the Speculative Society in Edinburgh. There was nothing elaborate in his composition, or imposing in his language, no rhetorical art in the structure of his periods, or the cadences of his sentences. Still, he was an agreeable and fascinating speaker; perhaps succeeding because he never thought of success, or aimed at it. It was not his habit to commit his lectures to writing. Possessed of a powerfully retentive memory, he had no difficulty, with the aid of some brief notes, in preserving the lucid arrangement of his topic, which he had previously settled in his mind. He never read a lecture but once, and he never repeated the experiment. The reading was irksome to him, and the previous writing more so. He returned to the method which was best suited to his powers, and in which, with his copiousness of knowledge and facility of elocution, he was certain of the success he desired, namely to convey to the mind of others, through the medium of simple, clear, forcible language, the luminous conceptions which he had formed in his own. In nothing did he show his contempt for vulgar display, and his high sense of duty, more than in his style of lecturing. His object was singly to instruct his audience, never for one moment to parade his own acquirements or ingenuity. He might have attracted more applause by discussing conflicting theories, amazed his hearers with brilliant speculation, or overwhelmed them with extent of erudition. But he never forgot that the province of the teacher is to enlighten, not to dazzle; and he also considered that theories and systems are the proper study for the closet, while practical information (particularly in subjects like surgery and medicine) is best communicated by the lectures of practical and experienced men. If, as a medical lecturer, he particularly excelled in any department, it was in delineating the features of disease from its small and scarcely perceptible beginnings, through its various phases and variations, either to recovery or dissolution. Here his graphic powers have never been surpassed. He presented to his audience a picture so faithful, so accurate, so vivid, that they almost fancied the ghastly phenomena of each malady were bodily before their eyes. For this power he was indebted not only to the vast extent of his anatomical researches, to which no man of his time had devoted himself so ardently, but also to the habit of keeping a minute record daily of every case that came under his personal observation. As a lecturer Colles was extremely popular; his style and language were simple and fluent, and partook more of the conversational character than of the didactic lessons of a teacher. In referring to writers with a view to strengthening a point of current testimony, or to overturning some absurd reasoning, or dangerous practice by some surgeon, or, rather, "writer on surgery", as he used to phrase it, his manner was warm and impressive and if he considered the point too absurd for serious argument, he indulged sometimes in a peculiar, quiet, caustic humour, scarcely less convincing than a critical analysis, but perhaps in better taste, because more appropriate. In his pleasantries there was a *utility*—in that they were worth more than the laugh-current, and when all was over the joke was not remembered without the maxim with which it was incorporated.

Colles never hesitated to tell his students of his own shortcomings: "8th September, 1799. A man came into the long ward with his arm badly wounded by glass. I was very cool, seeing at one view what actually might be necessary. So far I was pleased, but when the nurses and other attendants seemed to be too slow or to commit an error, then I was entirely too hasty and too anxious for them to hurry." A week later he was to write: "This day I removed a cancer. My anxiety for my own character was the predominant sensation at the commencement of the operation, but this gradually wore off and I soon felt for the success of the operation as if it had been a child of my own, or rather I felt as if I performed some piece of

mechanical work and was anxious for its success. My anxiety
at the beginning of the operation was greater than I wish it
to be on any future occasion, but on the whole I was well
pleased that my state of mind had been such as it was." A
year later he wrote: "Having shown you the manner in which
amputation should be performed, it will be in conformity with
the plan I have laid down to disclose to you those steps of the
operation in which I have erred from confusion, hurry, ignorance, or inadvertency. The first, and indeed a very capital error,
occurred in my application of the tourniquet, for the tourniquet
compress had not been applied with sufficient firmness, so that,
when the patient brought her body more erect the compress
was thrown off the artery"—and so he proceeds, pointing out
the errors to be avoided. Throughout his entire career as a
clinical teacher he lost no opportunity of frankly admitting his
blunders and making them the means of instructing his pupils.
The following anecdote is characteristic:—A patient in Dr.
Steevens' Hospital died after having been treated by Colles
for stricture of the rectum, by the introduction of a bougie.
Death had been unexpected. At the post-mortem examination
a malignant stricture was found, and below it a ragged opening
through the coats of the bowel into the peritoneum. The resident surgeon, when showing the specimen to Colles, took some
pains to explain that it was probably by extension of the
ulceration that the opening had been formed. "It is below the
stricture", said Colles. "Give me the bougie". The bougie,
having been produced, he passed its tip into the hole. "It fits
exactly," he said, and then he added, turning to his class,
"Gentlemen, it is no use mincing the matter, I caused the
patient's death," and then, without another word, and amidst
the absolute silence of his class, he walked out of the theatre.
Little wonder that his students trusted him utterly; few men in
that generation, or indeed in any other, have had the moral
courage to admit to their mistakes.

It is not surprising that Colles did not write much; the
wonder, on the contrary, is that he found time to make so many
additions as he did to medical literature. What leisure for
recreation, much less for study, is it possible for a surgeon in a
large practice to command? In fact the difficulty of dedicating

any portion of the day to the labour of composition is in direct proportion to the abundance of materials resulting from the range of observation and extent of experience. Colles was remarkable for the close attention which he devoted to every case that came before him, exhibiting any novel or striking feature, and in cases of such a description he was totally regardless of his pecuniary interests; but it was not often that he was able to extract from his practice the time that authorship requires. Nevertheless, he has left behind him some valuable contributions to medical science. As an author his language is correct, strong and explicit. He strove rather to express his ideas than to aim at eloquence or show. The simplicity of his language gives a kind of classical elegance united with a profound acuteness. He reasoned by analogy and induction from established facts. He never confused his reader with uncertain hypotheses founded on shifting principles. His cautiousness has been interpreted by some as showing lack of speculative power, and of ability to formulate those hypotheses which are so essential for extending the bounds of knowledge. We must remember, however, what a deceptive guide analogy often is in scientific reasoning and argument. We, his successors today, can well afford to be generous in our assessment, and to hope that our lack of speculative powers on the nature of carcinoma, for example, will be treated kindly by those to whom we pass the torch. Colles was the keen observer of all that passed before his eyes. His advance was made step by step, and there never were any of those flights of imagination by which genius changes the aspect of science. He recorded his observations on the good effect of mercury in certain diseases of the nervous system, as follows:

"I shall refrain from offering any theory, or attempt an explanation, of the modus operandi of mercury in this class of disease; partly because we are totally unable to do so in reference to those diseases in which its influence is still more marked and obvious, and in which its power over disease is almost certain, and unerring, or specific; but principally I abstain from offering any theoretical observations whatsoever because the class of diseases to which I have alluded are, as regards their pathology, involved in deep obscurity."

In the year 1811 Colles published the first part of *Surgical Anatomy*, a work of considerable industry and merit. It is a matter of general regret that he was never able to complete the second part. He deserves honour for having not only cultivated this important branch of the science, but having, by this publication, set an example which encouraged and stimulated others to its prosecution. The volume contains an accurate description of some of the most important and complex regions of the body, especially of femoral hernia, where his views were original, and his book deserves additional interest from a luminous exposition of his views upon the general subject of medical education. His account of the ligation of the subclavian artery for aneurysm is pregnant with interest, and it is impossible to read this brief paper without being struck as much by the modesty as by the ability of the writer. These operations, though unsuccessful, are recorded in the simplest and most laconic language, without the least assumption of merit or parade of discovery. Colles was distinguished at a very early period of life as a masterly operator. He was bold and enterprising, but at the same time steady, cool and dexterous, rapid without hurry, always prepared for sudden emergencies, and singularly fertile in resource. Of Colles' famous paper *On the fracture of the carpal extremity of the radius* Sir D'Arcy Power wrote: "Thus, with 1528 words and at the age of forty-one, Colles secured for himself a permanent name in surgery. It must be observed that his account is strictly clinical, for he had no opportunity of making a pathological examination of the injury." Colles' paper on club feet in infants has been overlooked by the profession, and the simple splints which he described for that deformity bear a striking resemblance to those now in use. His description of the peculiar enlargement of the inguinal lymph nodes is probably the first clinical account of *lymphogranuloma inguinale*. His description of the enlargement of axillary lymph nodes in carcinoma of the breast is as complete as any written today.

In politics Mr. Colles was a liberal. He held his political

opinions, as he did all others, with modest firmness, but without the faintest tinge of violence or party fanaticism. He was not one of those who sue for favours and when, in the year 1839, his claims as undisputed head of his profession in Ireland were overlooked, he was neither offended nor disturbed. The body of the profession, however, not only in Ireland, but, to their honour be it said, in England also, expressed their surprise and dissatisfaction. Sir Astley Cooper was one of the foremost in doing so. He bore witness to the general opinion of the profession in the British Empire, and declared that although Mr. Colles had achieved honour for himself far beyond what any government could bestow, nevertheless he was the legitimate channel through which to decorate in Ireland the profession to which he belonged. This opinion was so generally entertained and so strongly expressed as to reach the ears of the dispensers of patronage. They acknowledged their mistake, and strove to repair it. A baronetcy was offered and its acceptance more than once pressed on Mr. Colles. He, however, firmly but modestly, declined the proffered distinction. "If," he said, "it had been offered to him in the first instance, he should have considered it due to his profession to accept it; but that, for himself personally, such distinctions had no attraction, and that in consequence of the distribution he intended to make of his property amongst his children, a hereditary title would be an inconvenient honour." His family and descendants may point with just and honourable pride to the unadorned name of Abraham Colles, and boast that they are sprung from one who merited a title but declined it.

We take leave of this good tempered and good humoured man, surrounded by his students in the crowded out-patient department of Dr. Steevens' Hospital, when a confused old lady addressed him thus, "You are Mr. Collis, aren't you?" (referring to Maurice Collis, respected surgical contemporary and deeply religious man). "No, madam, you are mistaken." "You are seeking *Collis the Good:* I am *Colles the Great!*"

William Stokes gives us a very complete medical record of the final years and terminal illness of Colles. For some two years before he retired from the College chair of surgery in 1836, Colles had frequent attacks of gout in its ordinary form, and also chronic bronchitis. During these attacks, dyspnoea and palpitation were the prominent symptoms, but the disease always used to yield to small bleedings, followed by the exhibition of blue pill and Dover's powder. He was also occasionally affected with erysipelas of the face; and it was observed that the erysipelatous and gouty attacks were accompanied and followed by a suspension or diminution of the affections of the chest. In the session of 1836 he felt that after every lecture he was slightly feverish and that langour and debility followed; and under these circumstances, Professor Harrison felt it to be his duty to urge strongly on Colles the necessity of resigning the chair, which he had so long and so ably filled. He was attended by Dr. Cheyne, and after Dr. Cheyne's retirement, by Dr. John Crampton and Professor Harrison. The attacks of bronchitis recurred from time to time, and Dr. Crampton continued the practice of small bleedings, and on all occasions with the most marked benefit. He was bled about twelve times, but the operation was always somewhat difficult, and he at last adopted the practice of local bleedings for the relief of the attacks. Between these attacks of illness, Colles continued his duties at Dr. Steevens' Hospital and also managed some private practice with his son William, now helping him out in both. In 1840 Stokes was consulted on account of a dyspnoeic attack, when cupping and other means were employed, and Colles was soon to resume his professional labours. But the illness recurred, accompanied by gout in the ankles and in one knee, and when he showed signs of some improvement, he was advised to resign his hospital appointment in 1841, and go abroad for a complete change of air and for a more decided mental rest. Colles then went to Switzerland with his daughters, and he wrote home of his great delight in the improvement of his powers. On his return to London he was seen by several professional friends and was recommended carefully to abstain from all unnecessary muscular exertion. On returning to Dublin he decided to reside at Kingstown and for some time was under the care of Sir Henry Marsh. He now had oedema and enlargement of the liver, and thought that his Dublin colleagues had made an error as to the question of valvular disease, and that had this affection been sooner recognised, his treatment would have been different, and that the step of sending him to travel was a mistaken one. But Stokes, Marsh, Harrison and William Colles had long before come to the conclusion that the case was one of a weakened and dilated heart, with chronic bronchitis, and they never observed any unequivocal signs of disease of the heart valves; and this view, at post-mortem examination later, was found to be correct. Oedema, liver enlargement, anasarca, and diminution of urine occurred, but were usually relieved by the use of mercury, followed by ordinary diuretics.

For several years Colles had enjoyed the intimacy of Dr. Charles Dickinson, Lord Bishop of Meath, by whom his sons had been educated, and he had always taken much pleasure in the conversation of that pious and worthy man. During the early stages of his malady, having upon one occasion felt a desire to receive the sacrament at his own house, and being unable to attend public worship, he wrote to the bishop expressing his wish to have the rite administered by the hands of a friend with whom he had often discussed the truths of Christianity. On that day (12th July 1842) that should have brought Dr. Dickinson to his side, upon the mission of religion and friendship, Colles received the tidings of his untimely end.

In the autumn of 1842 Colles, having recovered from one of his severe attacks, stated to Stokes his conviction that his end was approaching, and that though by the aid of medicine his symptoms had been so often relieved, the time must soon arrive when remedies must fail, and with all the calmness of a true philosopher, and all the zeal of a great physician, he requested that a post-mortem examination of his body should be made by Dr. Robert William Smith in the presence of his medical attendants; observing that he trusted the knowledge thus obtained would not be useless, and that he felt sure the observations would be made with accuracy and reported with truth. Soon after this he wrote the following letter to Professor Harrison, which all right-minded men will read with feelings of emotion and gratitude:

October 22nd, 1842

My Dear Robert,

I think it may be of some benefit, not only to my own family, but to society at large, to ascertain by examination the exact seat and nature of my last disease. I am sure you will grant my request, that you will see this be *carefully* and *early* done. The parts to which I would direct particular attention are the heart and lungs, a small hernia immediately above the umbilicus, and the swelling in the right hypochondrium. From the similarity of the Rev. P. Roe's case with mine, I suppose there is some connection between the swelling of the hypochondrium and the diseased state of the heart.

Yours truly, dear Robert,

A. Colles.

This letter was the last great act of Colles' medical career, the last evidence of his unchanging devotion to that science on which he had already bestowed so many excellent gifts. That he was animated by a pure desire to advance medicine is obvious, and it is interesting to reflect that at that time the respective heads of the medical (Robert Perceval) and surgical professions in Dublin set the example of bequeathing their mortal remains for the benefit of that science for which they had laboured so long and so successfully.

But the final termination of the disease was more remote than he had anticipated. The urgency of the symptoms having been removed, Colles continued using small doses of mercury and regained a state of health which was indeed a surprise to himself. He had a good appetite, he drank wine, took carriage exercises, and even attended to professional business in his house. In addition to the blue pill, the diuretic which answered best was a combination of the infusion of digitalis with ammonia, ether, and tincture of cantharides. In the autumn of 1843, symptoms commenced which ushered in the closing scene. He was now obliged to remain in his chair or propped up in bed, and his calmness and fortitude under continued suffering was the only support of his sorrowing and anxious family and friends. He died on 1st December, 1843, preserving his strength of mind to the last moment of his life.

A member of his family wrote: "On the 1st December Abraham said he would not outlive two days. He was calm and cheerful, he gave directions as coolly as if he were ordering his carriage for some ordinary occasion, collected his family about him, conversed on ordinary subjects, and at seven in the evening desired them to order tea in his room that he might see one more cheerful meal. He looked happy when he saw them about the table, encouraged conversation, and placing his arm around his poor wife who sat beside him on the sofa, pressed her to his heart and expired so gently that until a loud cry from his eldest son announced the fact, she was not aware of it."

A post-mortem examination was performed by Dr. Robert William Smith in the presence of Sir Henry Marsh, Professor Robert Harrison, and Dr. William Stokes, and the findings were communicated to the Pathological Society of Dublin on December 9th, 1843 by Dr. Smith. These were chronic bronchitis, a fibrotic left lung, a dilated and fatty heart, without valvular disease.

When the news of his death reached the city, all the medical schools in Dublin closed as a mark of respect. The funeral procession was one of the largest ever witnessed in the capital. Merrion Row and the north and west sides of St. Stephen's Green were impassable with mourners and their carriages. The fellows of the Royal College of Physicians walked from the house of their president in Merrion Square, and were joined by members of the Apothecaries Company; likewise the Judiciary, headed by the Master of the Rolls, took their places in the long procession. As the hearse passed the Royal College of Surgeons the gates were thrown open, the president, council, members and licentiates pouring out in procession, all leaving their carriages to follow on foot on the long walk to Mount Jerome Cemetery. The chief mourners who followed the hearse were the five sons of the deceased; his brothers-in-law, the Rev. Thomas Ottiwell Moore, D.D. and Professor Robert Harrison; his sons-in-law, Major James Harrison and James Arthur Wall; and his cousin, Edward Richard Purefoy Colles.

Lives of great men all remind us, wrote Longfellow in those all too memorable lines,

> *We* can make *our* lives sublime,
> And departing, leave behind us
> Footprints on the sands of time.

APPENDIX 1

ABRAHAM COLLES

Curriculum Vitae

1773, 23rd July	Born at Millmount, Co. Kilkenny.
1780–1790	Educated at Mr. William Lindsay's Preparatory School, Kilkenny, and at Kilkenny College.
1790. 1st September	Entered Trinity College, University of Dublin, as a student of Arts.
1790, 15th September	Indentured to Philip Woodroffe, Resident Surgeon at Dr. Steevens' Hospital for his clinical training.
1790–1795	Registered Pupil of the Surgeons' School of the Royal College of Surgeons in Ireland. Attended two courses of lectures, Chemistry (Robert Perceval) and Practice of Medicine (Stephen Dickson) at the School of Physic, Trinity College, Dublin, and one clinical session at the House of Industry.
1795, April	Graduated B.A. at University of Dublin.
1795, 24th September	Granted "Letters Testimonial" or Licence of the Royal College of Surgeons in Ireland.
1795 (September)– 1797 (June)	In Edinburgh.
1797, June	Graduated M.D., Edinburgh University.
1797, June–November	In London.
1797, November	Returned to Dublin.
1797–1799	In private practice in Dublin. Private teaching of Anatomy and Surgery.
1799, 26th July	Appointed Resident Surgeon, Dr. Steevens' Hospital.
1799, 4th November	Elected a Member of the Royal College of Surgeons in Ireland.
1800, 6th January	Elected an Assistant at the College.
1801, 5th January	Elected a Censor of the College.
1802, 4th January	Elected President of the College.

1803, October	Appointed Surgeon to Cork Street Fever Hospital.
1804, 4th September	Appointed Professor of Anatomy and Physiology and Professor of Surgery at the Surgeons' School of the Royal College of Surgeons in Ireland.
1807, 27th April	Married Sophia, dau. of Rev. Jonathan Cope, Rector of Ahascragh, Co. Galway.
1811	Published *A Treatise on Surgical Anatomy*, Dublin.
1813, 29th January	Appointed Assistant Surgeon, Dr. Steevens' Hospital.
1814	Paper on "Fracture of carpal extremity of radius" published in *Edinb. med. and surg. Jour.*
1815	Paper on "The operation of tying the subclavian artery" published in *Edinb. med. and surg. Jour.*
1819, 22nd November	Appointed Governor of Dr. Steevens' Hospital.
1820, 3rd November	Appointed Consulting Surgeon to the Lying-in Hospital (Rotunda).
1824	Published *Practical Precepts on injuries of the Head*, Dublin.
1827, August	Resigned the chair of Anatomy and Physiology (but retained chair of Surgery).
1830	Elected President of the Royal College of Surgeons in Ireland for the second time.
1832	Graduated M.A. at University of Dublin.
1836, 19th September	Resigned the chair of Surgery, at the Surgeons' School.
1837	Published *Practical Observations on the Venereal Disease and on the use of Mercury*, London.
1838	Presented with an Address by the College and also with a piece of silver plate. His portrait painted by Martin Cregan, P.R.H.A. and his bust sculptured by Kirk, were placed in the College.
1841, 19th August	Resigned appointment of assistant surgeon at Dr. Steevens' Hospital.
1843, 1st December	Died at his home, 21 St. Stephen's Green, Dublin, and was buried at Mount Jerome Cemetery.

APPENDIX 2

CHILDREN OF ABRAHAM COLLES AND SOPHIA COLLES, née COPE

MARY ANNE = Lt. Col. James Harrison, Madras Artillery (1832)
b. 24th July 1808
d. 17th November 1850

WILLIAM (of St. Stephen's Green) = Penelope, d. of Cadwallader Waddy, Co. Wexford (1st September 1859)
Surgeon in Ordinary to the Queen in Ireland.
b. 2nd July 1809   B.A. Trinity College, Dublin, 1831.
M.B. 1841.   M.D. 1865.
President of the Royal College of Surgeons in Ireland, 1863-4.
Regius Professor of Surgery, University of Dublin, 1875.
d. 18th June 1892 (buried Mt. Jerome Cemetery)

HENRY JONATHAN COPE = Elizabeth, d. of John Mayne of Dublin (1845)
b. 24th June 1810.   B.A. Trinity College, Dublin, 1831.
Barrister 1832.
Principal Taxing Master of the Courts of Chancery and Common Law in Ireland.
d. 25th or 26th December 1877 (buried Mt. Jerome Cemetery)

FRANCES MARIA
b. 2nd October 1811
d. 10th May 1812

SOPHIA—unmarried.
b. 25th October 1813
d. 11th November 1899

ABRAHAM = Anna Countess, d. of Francis Hopkins, J.P., Co. Cork.
Known as Abraham of Ballyfallon, Co. Meath.
b. 23rd February 1815   B.A. Trinity College, Dublin, 1836.   J.P.
d. July 1879

THOMAS
b. 20th February 1817
d. 28th March 1829

RICHARD = Frances Ann, d. of J. Wilmett (Advocate) of Bordeaux, France. (10th February 1841).
b. 5th March 1818   B.A. Trinity College, Dublin, 1841.
Called to English Bar, 1842.
Went to Australia, 1852.
M.A. Melbourne University, 1861.
Sheriff of Castlemaine, Victoria, 1854-1883.
d. 12th December 1883 (in Australia)

FRANCES JANE = James Arthur Wall, of Knockrigg, Co. Wicklow Q.C., J.P., County Court Judge, Co. Tipperary.
b. 8th October 1819
d. (?)

MARIA JANE COPE—unmarried.
b. 19th December 1820

GRAVES CHAMNEY = (1) Mary Anne, d. of Robert Harrison, M.D. Dublin.
(2) Seremma, d. of Rev. John Blower.
b. 15th March 1823   B.A. Trinity College, Dublin, 1844.
M.A. 1865.
Admitted a Solicitor Trinity term 1845.
d. 4th August 1887
d. 1892

APPENDIX 3

COLLES FAMILY RECORDS

1. Some notes concerning the Family of Colles, by Richard Colles, 1927.   Typescript.

2. The Pedigree of the Family of Colles in Ireland, by J. H. Glascott, J.P. and Rev. W. Morris Colles, D.D. For private circulation. London, 1886.   Spottiswoode & Co., Printers.

3. Records of the Family of Colles, by Richard William Colles (Ramsay Colles). For private circulation. Dublin, 1892.   Charles Chambers, Printers.

4. Notes on the Family of Colles of Leigh, by Dr. J. A. Purefoy Colles, 1872.   Typescript.

5. The Family of Colles in Ireland, being Chapter XXVIII of *In Castle and Court House* by Ramsay Colles. London, 1911.

6. Colles Pedigrees in British Museum.
   Harley MS. 1566, fol. 141.
   Harley MS. 1196, ff. 15, 23.
   Harley MS. 1110, ff. 109–109b.

7. Worcester City Archives.
   Documents of Grant of Administration to Margaret Colles, widow of late William Colles of Lusley, who died in 1596. She signs with her mark, as does the other Administrator, William Coles (?)

8. Original correspondence of Abraham Colles and his Family in possession of:
   Ronald M. Colles.
   Sir Dudley Colles.
   Mrs. George Lucas.
   Christopher Colles McCready.

9. Colles Family History and Pedigree with two contemporary documents 1728 and 1751, and letters of William Colles of Abbeyvale.

Prim. MSS. No. 86–87 and 88–89. Public Record Office, Dublin.

10. Ancestry of Christopher Colles in Ireland, By Christopher J. Colles, M.D.

Journal of the American Irish Historical Society. 1931 : 29 : 67

11. Colles family records in *The Parish of Taney* by F. E. Ball and E. Hamilton. Dublin, 1895.

Hodges, Figgis & Co. Ltd.

APPENDIX 4

COLLES Harl., 1566, fol. 141, etc.

ARMS.—Quarterly of six: Gules, a chevron argent between three lion's heads erased, Or, COLLES; 2, Per fess, or, and argent, three estoiles sable, HIGH; 3, AZURE, a *fleur-de-lis* in chief argent, and two trefoils in base, Or, within a bordure engrailed of the last, PALMER; 4, Argent, two bars vert, HERTHULL or HARTHILL; 5, Gules, a bend cottised between six martlets. Or, COTTON; 6, Per chevron crenellée sable and argent, three mullets counter changed, CHEESMAN.

CREST.—A sea-pie, with wings endorsed, sable platée, on a dolphin, lying on its back proper.

RICHARD COLLES, of Powick, in the Parish of Suckley,=MARGARETT, da. of THOM. HALL, of........in com. Worcester. in com. Worcester, 26 H.C.

ISSABELL, dau. of Richard Turber-=WILLIAM COLLES, of Brawnfford Court, in=ALLICE, dau. of Rompney, of........in com. ville, 1 wiffe. com. Worcester. Worster, 2 wiffe.

1. WILLIAM, ob. s.p. 2. WILLIAM COLLES, of Long...=MARGARET JOANE, VX. dau. of... MARGARET VX... ELIZABETH 1 VX [? Longdon] in com. Worster Hich, of— Vaughan......in com. Burnfford, of com. Stokes, 2 to sepul. Ibidem, 1558. Gloucester. Worster. Parsonns.

JOANE, dau. of Robert=1. EDMOND COLLES,=ANNE, dau. of.....Town- ELIZABETH VX., Law- 4. JOHN COLLES, of Somerville. of com. of Lye, in com. Wor- send, 2 wiffe. rence Rompney, of Hattfield, in com. Warwick, 1 wiffe. cester. Kingswick. Hertfford.

MARY, dau. of Jerom Palmer, of=WILLIAM COLLES, of Lye=ELIZABETH, dau. of.....Lord JANE VX.....Daunteshey, of Kentishtowne, in com. Midlesex, Cromwell, 2. wiffe. ......in com, Herefford. sole heire to her father.

2. JOHN COLLES=MARY, dau. of...... 3. THOMAS COLLES Borough. 4.JEROMY COLLES.

1. EDMOND COLLES,=MARTHA, dau. of Wm. Tirwhitt, 2. JOHN COLLES. 3. THOMAS COLLES. 4. ROBERT COLLES. 1619. of Kettleby, in com. Lincon.

1. WILLIAM COLLES.

ANNE VX. Sir Walter Leveson, of Wolver- JANE VX. Raffe Selby, of Barwick. MARY VX. Francis Blount, of Astley, hampton, in com. Stafford. in com. Worster.

2. EDMOND COLLES=ELIZABETH, dau. of......Fisher.

3 RICHARD COLLES=ELIZABETH, dau. of......Corningsby.

SUSAN VX. Sir Edmond Hare-well, Knt. of the Bath.

JOHN COLLES=MARY, dau. of......Corningsby.

GRACE VX. Ed-mond Atwood.

MARY VX. Thom. Rowlandal's Stayner.

WALTER COLLES

WILLIAM COLLES

EDMOND COLLES

3. WILLIAM COLLES=MARGERY, dau. of Hum-ffrey Pakington, of Lon-don. Marchant.

ALICE VX. Raffe Odell, of T'inifford, in com. Nort'iampton.

JANE VX.......Ruding, of ......in com. Worseter.

VRSULA VX. William Hawes, of Solihull, in com. Warwick.

2. MICHELL COLLES, of Brad-well, in com. Buckingham, 1619, and of Hampton Arden, in com. Warwick.

=MARY, dau. of Edward Graunt, of Snitterffeld, in com. War-wick.

ANNE VX. Ric. Pitcher, of Crad-ley, in com. Herefford.

MARY VX. Raffe Vnderhill, of Stouley, in com. Warwick.

ANNE COLLES VX. William Colles, of London, Marchant.

CATHERIN VX. William Bustard, of Adderbury in com. Oxon.

ISABELL VX. Thomas Pointe (?) of Mal-lets, in Stony Strat-ford, in Co. War-wick.

VRSULA 1. Francis Hall. 2. to John Joanes. 3. to Arthur Bagshaw.

JOYCE VX. 1. Richard Bluddy. 2. to Silves-ter Robbins.

JOHN COLLES

JOANE VX. Richard Judd, of Elmedon, in com. Warwick.

1. HUMFFREY COLLES, of the Middle Temple, 1619.

=MARY, dau. of William Chamb'lyn, 4th son of Sir Leonard Chamb'lyn, of Sherborne, in com. Oxon.

1. WILL'M COLLES, 21 yere old. 1619.

2. MICHELL.

3. HUMFFREY. s.p.

4. JOHN.

MARGARET. s.p.

MARGERY. s.p.

MARY.

APPENDIX 5

COLLES FAMILY PEDIGREE (in part) IN IRELAND

WILLIAM COLLES of Doughill, near Athlone. (1585–1621)

JOB COLLES (1607–1655) — one daughter

WILLIAM COLLES of Skinner's Row (now Christchurch Place) Dublin (1610–1678)

Rev. CHRISTOPHER COLLES (?–d. 1724)

CHARLES COLLES of Maghermore, Co. Sligo (1616–1685)

ROSE COLLES (b. 1613?)

WILLIAM COLLES of Kilcollen (1648–1719)

CHARLES COLLES Skinner's Row (now Christchurch Pl.) (b. 1651–?)

BARRY COLLES (1697–1785) — one daughter

WILLIAM COLLES of Abbeyvale (1702–1770)

RICHARD COLLES of Dublin (1707–1749)

CHRISTOPHER COLLES of Dublin and New York (1739–1816)

WILLIAM COLLES of Millmount (1745–1779)

RICHARD COLLES of 119 (now 135) St. Stephen's Green, and Prospect, Co. Dublin. Barrister. (1747–1816)

JOHN COLLES of Dublin and New York. (1751–1807). Bookseller.

WILLIAM COLLES (2nd) of Millmount. Surgeon. (1772–1849)

ABRAHAM COLLES Surgeon. (1773–1843)

RICHARD COLLES of Riverview. (1774–1849)

RACHEL COLLES (1776–1864)

EDWARD R. COLLES Barrister. (1798–1883)

WILLIAM H. G. COLLES (1803–1880)

WILLIAM COLLES Surgeon. (1809–1892)

HENRY J. C. COLLES. (1810–1877)

WILLIAM COLLES of Pubna (1811–1873)

JOHN A. PUREFOY COLLES (1835–1873)

GODDARD R. P. COLLES (1838–1895)

ALEXANDER COLLES of Millmount (1815–1876)

RICHARD COLLES of Gaya (1827–1868)

EDWARD G. T. COLLES (1851–1911)

ABRAHAM COLLES (1847–1912)

JOHN MAYNE COLLES (1858–1922)

RICHARD COLLES (1844–1929)

RICHARD W. COLLES (Ramsay Colles) (1862–1919)

RONALD M. COLLES

A. C. COLLES

SIR DUDLEY COLLES

APPENDIX 6

THE COPE FAMILY TREE

Vice-Chamberlain to Catharine Parr, Knighted by Edward VI, Sheriff for Oxfordshire and Berks, 1548.

SIR ANTHONY COPE, Kt. = **JANE,** dau. of Matthew Crews of Pynne, Devon.

ANNE = Kenelm Digby of Dry-stoke, Co. Rutland.

EDWARD COPE of Hanwell, Co. Oxford = **ELIZABETH,** dau. and h. of Walter Mohan, of Wallaston, Northamptonshire.

SIR WALTER COPE of Kensington, Master of the Court of Wards *temp.* James I, and a Chamberlain of the Exchequer: built Holland House.

ANNE, dau. of Sir Wm. Paston, Kt. of Paston, Norfolk. = **SIR ANTHONY COPE,** bart. = **FRANCES,** dau. of Rowland Lytton, Esq. of Knebsworth, Co. Hertford: (1st wife). High Sheriff for Cc. of Oxford 1581 and 1590. Represented Banbury in Parliament in seven Parliaments *temp.* Elizabeth, and the Co. of Oxford *temp.* James I: Knighted by Queen Elizabeth, and a baronet by James I, 29th June 1611.

RICHARD COPE = **ANNE WALTER,** Settled in Ireland. Sister of Sir William Walter of Wimbledon, Surrey.

Sir WILLIAM COPE, bart. = **ELIZABETH,** dau. of Sir Geo. Chaworth of Wiverton, Notts.

ANTHONY COPE = **ELIZABETH,** dau. of Captain Sheffield of Vaughal. Settled in Ireland.

ANTHONY COPE of Portadown, Co. Armagh. d. Aug. 1642. = **JANE,** dau. of Right Rev. Thomas Moigne, Lord Bishop of Kilmore and Ardagh, app. 1612, d. 31st December 1640. buried in St. Patrick's Cathedral.

HARRY COPE of Laughgall, Co. Armagh. =

ELIZABETH = Very Rev. **ANTHONY COPE,** Dean of Elphin. app. 28th August 1683, resigned 1700. d. February 1705-

HENRY COPE, M.D. of = **MARY PAGE** Dublin.

HENRY COPE of Laughgall.

Rev. **JONATHAN COPE,** Rector of Ahascragh, Co. Galway. b. 1727. =

SOPHIA = **ABRAHAM COLLES, M.D.** of Dublin.
b. 4th January 1782   b. 23rd July 1773.
m. 25th April 1807   d. 1st December 1843.
d. 21st February 1858.

[Reproduced by courtesy of Ronald M. Colles.]

APPENDIX 7

ABRAHAM COLLES—PUBLICATIONS

De Venaesectione, M.D. Thesis, Univ. Edinb. (1797)

A Treatise on Surgical Anatomy (Part the First)
  Gilbert and Hodges (1811), Dublin.
  Maxwell, J. (1820), Philadelphia.
  Carey, J. and Lea (Second American Edition) (1931), Philadelphia.

On the Fracture of the carpal extremity of the radius.
  Edinb. med. and surg. J. (1814) *10* : 182

On the operation of tying the Subclavian Artery.
  Edinb. med. and surg. J. (1815) *11* : 1

On the distortion termed Varus or Club Feet.
  Dubl. Hosp. Reports. (1817) *1* : 175

On the cause of the disease Trismus Nascentium.
  Dubl. Hosp. Reports. (1817) *1* : 285

On a disease of the Lymphatic Glands of the Groin attended with
  peculiar symptoms.
  Dubl. Hosp. Reports. (1818) *2* : 268

Fracture of the Neck of the Femur.
  Dubl. Hosp. Reports. (1818) *2* : 334

Fatal consequences resulting from slight wounds received in Dissection.
  Dubl. Hosp. Reports. (1822) *3* : 203

Practical Precepts on injuries of the Head.
  Hodges and McArthur (1824), Dublin.
  The Lancet (1825) 7 : 210

On Tetanus—Lecture delivered in Theatre, R.C.S.I.
  The Lancet (1825) *10* : 37

On Hydrophobia—Lecture delivered in Theatre R.C.S.I.
  The Lancet (1825) *10* : 73

Second communication relative to the fatal consequences which
  result from slight wounds received in Dissection.
  Dubl. Hosp. Reports. (1827) *4* : 240

Practical observations upon certain diseases of the Anus and Rectum.
   Dubl. Hosp. Reports. (1830) 5 : 131

Practical observations on Venereal Disease and on the use of
   Mercury.
   Sherwood, Gilbert and Piper (1837), London.
   Waldie, A. (1837), Philadelphia.
   German Edition (1839), Hamburg.

Observations on some morbid afflictions of the Nail of the Great
   Toe.
   Dubl. J. med. and chem. Sci. (1848) 23 : 240

Lectures on the Theory and Practice of Surgery, by the late Abraham
   Colles.
   Edited by Simon McCoy, F.R.C.S.I.
   Dublin Medical Press. (1844) Vol. XI and XII.
   Reprinted Machen, S. J. (1844) Vol. I. Dublin.
              Machen, S. J. (1845) Vol. II. Dublin.
              Barrington and Haswell. (1845). Philadelphia.

Selections from the unpublished MSS. of the late Abraham Colles.
   Edited by his son, William Colles, F.R.C.S.I.

1.	Tetanus	*Dubl. Quart. J. med. Sci.*				(1853) 15 : 280
2.	Injuries of the Head	,,	,,	,,	,,	(1853) 16 : 55
3.	Surgical Diseases of the Neck and Throat	,,	,,	,,	,,	(1853) 16 : 290
4.	A Peculiar Disease of the Rectum.	,,	,,	,,	,,	(1854) 17 : 82
5.	On Varicose Veins	,,	,,	,,	,,	(1854) 18 : 28
6.	On Diseases and Injuries of Arteries.	,,	,,	,,	,,	(1855) 20 : 335
7.	On Diseases of the Urinary Organs.	,,	,,	,,	,,	(1856) 22 : 27
8.	On Diseases of the Genital Organs and Rectum, and on Brachial Aneurysm.	,,	,,	,,	,,	(1857) 23 : 374

APPENDIX 8

THE ABRAHAM COLLES ROOMS AND THE ABRAHAM COLLES LECTURES

The Abraham Colles Rooms

In 1948 two rooms in the ground floor of the Royal College of Surgeons in Ireland were designated the Abraham Colles Rooms, and included a stained glass window of the Colles arms, donated by Mr. T. O. Graham (President, R.C.S.I., 1942–44), who was a descendant of Rachel Colles—Abraham's sister.

The Abraham Colles Lectures

In 1956 the College, on the proposal of Mr. T. G. Wilson, Vice-President, decided to institute a series of post-graduate lectures, to be styled the Abraham Colles Lectures and to be given annually in the College. The roll of the distinguished lecturers now reads:

1956	Professor Charles Wells.
1957	Sir Eric William Riches.
1957	Mr. David Howard Patey.
1958	Dr. O. Theron Clagett.
1958	Professor Sir Walter Mercer.
1959	Mr. R. Vaughan Hudson.
1959	Sir Archibald H. McIndoe.
1960	Sir Stanford Cade.
1960	Mr. Ion Simson Hall.
1960	Professor Sir John Bruce.
1962	Professor Clarence Crafoord.
1963.	Mr. Harold C. Edwards.
1963	Mr. J. Angell James.
1964	Professor F. J. Gillingham.
1964	Dr. Herbert Conway.
1965	Lord Brock.
1966	Sir Henry Osmond-Clarke.
1967	Dr. Michael E. De Bakey.
1967	Dr. John Conley.
1968	Sir James Fraser.
1969	Mr. Geoffrey Bateman.
1970	Professor J. C. Goligher.
1972	Dr. George Zuidema.

REASONS

For Regulating the Practice of

𝔖urgery in the 𝔠ity of 𝔇ublin

By Making the SURGEONS a Distinct Society from
the Barbers, Peruke-Makers, &c.

*Humbly Offer'd to the Consideration of the LORDS Spiritual
and Temporal, and the Commons in Parliament Assembled.*

There is not any place where Surgery hath the least Reputation (except in this Kingdom) but every
Person professing that Art, is obliged to prove himself qualify'd before he is admitted to Practice.
　　The present Corporation in this City is composed of *Barbers, Surgeons, Apothecaries* and *Peruke-Makers*, which (instead of Encouraging the true Professors of *Surgery*) is a refuge for Empiricks,
Impudent Quacks, Women, and other Idle Persons, who quit the Trades to which they were bred,
and wherein they might be useful to the Commonwealth, to undertake a Profession whereof they
are entirely ignorant, to the ruine of their Fellow Subjects.
　　There is not any Person (tho of the most Infamous Character) who cannot obtain his Freedom
of the Corporation, by Vertue whereof, the meanest Brother assumeth the Liberty, and it is a sufficient
Recommendation for him to Practice *Surgery*, with as much Authority as the most Experienced
Surgeon.
　　There are in the Corporation at least Ten *Barbers, &c.* for one *Surgeon*, so that it is impossible
for the *Surgeons* to make any Regulation, because they must inevitably be out-voted by the Majority
of the others.
　　There is not the least Affinity between *Surgery, Peruke-Makeing*, and the Feat or Craft of *Barbery*, it
not being necessary for a *Surgeon* to know how to make a *Peruke* or *Cut Hair*, nor is it any part of
a *Barber's* or *Peruke-Makers* Trade, to perform any operation in *Surgery*.
　　It is requisite for a *Surgeon* (to arrive to a tolerable perfection in his Profession) to have a reasonable understanding of *Latin* and *Greek*; whereas a *Peruke-Maker* or a *Barber* may be Masters of their
Trades tho they are wholly illeterate.
　　Wherefore, It is Humbly offer'd to the Consideration of this Honourable Assembly, whether it
is not highly unreasonable and dangerous to the health of Her Majesty's good Subjects, that such
Barbers, &c. as take upon them (tho' not in the least qualified) to Practice *Surgery*, shou'd be allow'd
the same Priviledge therein, as *Surgeons* who have taken great pains to make themselves Masters
of the Art of *Surgery*, and whose Parents have been at great Expence to make them capable.

The Advantages which will necessarily arise from such a Regulation will be

The preservation of many Subjects lives, which are lost by the gross Errors, and the Barbarous
and Inhumane Practice of Impudent Ignorant Pretenders, of which there are too many Instances
which daily offer, to the great prejudice of the Publick, and discredit of the Profession.
　　It will encourage such persons as can afford to give their Children Learning sufficient for the
Profession, to breed them to it.
　　It will oblige Apprentices to be diligent and studious in the Profession, whereby the Kingdom
and Army will be supply'd with a succession of Experienced and Judicious Surgeons.
　　It will be an encouragement to Honest and Skilful Practitioners, to converse with greater freedom,
so as to improve the Art.
　　It is probable (that in some time) the Professors of Surgery in this Kingdom, may acquire such
a reputation, as may prevent Young Men's going into foreign Countreys to compleat their Studies.
　　Many other Reasons may be offer'd, but it is hoped that these may prove sufficient to make this
August Assembly sensible of the great benefit a due Regulation of the practice of Surgery will be
to the Publick, and to induce them to Enact such Laws as in their Wisdom shall be thought most
proper, to encourage the true Practice of Surgery in this Kingdom, and punish the abuse thereof.

Reproduced by courtesy of the National Library of Ireland.

APPENDIX 10

BIBLIOGRAPHY

(A) General:

Abernethy, John.
Surgical and Physiological Essays. London. 1797.
Surgical Observations. London. 1804.
Surgical observations on injuries of the head and on miscellaneous subjects. London. 1825.

Abraham, J. Johnston.
The Night Nurse. London. 1913.

Adams, Robert.
Cases of diseases of the heart accompanied with pathological observations.
Dubl. Hosp. Reports. 1827 : *4* : 353.

Alcock, Benjamin.
R. B. Todd's *Cyclopaedia of Anatomy and Physiology.* London. 1836 : *2* : 835.

Bennett, Edward Hallaran.
Fracture of the Metacarpal Bones.
Dubl. J. med. Sci. 1882 : *73* : 72.

Berry, Henry F.
The Ancient Corporation of Barber-Surgeons or Guild of St. Mary Magdalene.
Jour. Roy. Soc. Antiq. of Ireland. Dublin. 1903 : *33* : 217.

Bishop, W. J.
The Early History of Surgery. London. 1960.

Blacker, William.
Journal. Quoted in Maxwell's History of Trinity College, Dublin. 1946.

Carmichael, Richard.
Review of Colles' "Practical Observations on the Venereal Disease".
Dubl. J. med. Sci. 1837 : *34* : 25.

Cameron, Sir Charles A.
On the anatomical knowledge and original discoveries of Irish surgeons.
Dubl. J. med. Sci. 1885 : *80* : 453.
History of the Royal College of Surgeons in Ireland. 2nd Edit. Dublin. 1916.

Cheyne, John.
A case of apoplexy in which the fleshy part of the heart was converted into fat. *Dubl. Hosp. Reports.* 1818 : *2* : 216.
Essays on partial derangement of the mind in supposed connection with religion. Dublin. 1843.

Cleghorn, George.
Observations on the Epidemical Diseases of Minorca (1744–1749). London. 1751.
Index of an Annual Course of Lectures. Dublin. 1756.
Also see Lettsom's memoirs of J. Fothergill. London. 1786.

Cloncurry, Lord.
Personal Recollections on the Life and Times. . . Dublin. 1849.

Colles, Mr.
Diary of events 1685–1690.
Ormonde Papers H.M.C. 2nd series. *8* : 343.

Comrie, John D.
History of Scottish Medicine. 2nd Edit. London. 1932.

Cooper, Astley.
Surgical Essays. London. 1818.
A Treatise on Dislocations and on Fractures of the Joints. 3rd Edit. London. 1824.

Craig, Maurice.
Dublin 1660–1860. Dublin. 1969.

Crampton, John.
Medical Report. Dublin. 1819.

Crampton, Philip.
An outline of the History of Medicine and Surgery.
Dubl. J. med. Sci. 1839 : *14* : 504.

Croly, Henry Gray.
Hernia and Taxis.
Dubl. J. med. Sci. 1895 : *No. 283* : 1. 1895 : *No.* 284 : 97.

Curtis, Edmund.
A History of Ireland. London. 1936.

Dease, William.
Preface to Radical cure of Hydrocele. Dublin. 1782.
Observations on Wounds of the Head. Dublin. 1778.

Diday, P.
A Treatise on Syphilis in new born children and infants at the breast.
Translated by G. Whitley. London. 1859.

Doolin, William.
The Pathfinders. *Ir. J. med. Sci.* 1945 : *230* : 33.

Doolin, William—*continued*
   Wayfarers in Medicine. London. 1947.
   Dublin Surgery 100 years ago. *Ir. J. med. Sci.* 1949 : *279* : 97.
   Dublin's Surgeon–Anatomists. *Ann. R. Coll. Surg.* 1951 : *8* : 1.
Dublin Medical Press.
   Records of Medical Meetings and Speeches by Colles. 1839 : *1* :
      400. 1841 : *5* : 384.
Duncan, A. (Jun.)
   Medical Education. *Edinb. med. & surg. J.* 1827 : *27* : 368.
"Erinensis" (Dr. Herris Greene).
   The Lancet. 1823–1830.
"Eblanensis".
   Lond. Med. Gaz. 1828 : *1* : 533 & 828.
Foster, Sir Michael.
   Lectures on the History of Physiology. Cambridge. 1901.
Hutchinson, Johnathan.
   Syphilis. London. 1887.
Gamble, John.
   Sketches . . . . in Dublin and the north of Ireland. London. 1811.
Gilborne, John.
   The Medical Review . . . . Dublin. 1775.
Gogarty, Oliver St. John.
   As I was going down Sackville Street. London. 1937.
Graves, Robert James.
   Newly observed affection of the thyroid gland in females. *Lond.*
      med. & surg. Jour. (Renshaw volume). 1835 : 7 : 516.
   Clinical Lectures on the Practice of Medicine. 2nd Edit. Dublin.
      1848.
Green, John Richard.
   A Short History of the English People. London. 1882.
Guthrie, Douglas.
   A History of Medicine (1945). London. Thomas Nelson & Son.
Harrison, Robert.
   The Dublin Dissector. 5th Edit. Dublin. 1848.
Houston, John.
   Valves of the Rectum. *Dubl. Hosp. Reports.* 1830 : 5 : 158.
Jackson, Hughlings.
   Epileptiform seizures (unilateral) after an injury to the head.
      Med. Times and Hosp. Gaz. 1863 : 2 : 65.
Jacob, Arthur.
   An account of a membrane in the eye, now first described.
      Phil. Trans. 1819 : *109* : 300.

Jacob, Arthur—*continued*
  Observations respecting an ulcer of peculiar character which attacks the eyelids and other parts of the face. *Dubl. Hosp. Reports.* 1827 : *4* : 232.
Kirkpatrick, T. Percy C.
  History of the Medical School in Trinity College, Dublin. Dublin. 1912.
  Diary of an Irish Medical Student (1831–1837). *Dubl. J. med. Sci.* 1913 : *136* : 360.
  Index to papers on the History of Medicine. *Dubl. J. med. Sci.* 1916 : *3* : 302.
  Index to biographical notices. *Dubl. J. med. Sci.* 1916 : *142* : 110.
  History of Dr. Steevens' Hospital, Dublin. Dublin. 1924.
  The Schools of Medicine in Dublin in the nineteenth century. *Br. med. J.* 1933 : *1* : 109.
  Dr. Steevens' Hospital. *Med. Press and Circulr.* 1944 : *211* : 132.
Labatt, Samuel B.
  Review of Colles' paper. *Edinb. med. and surg. J.* 1819 : *15* : 216.
The Lancet.
  Editorials. 1833 : *2* : 79. 1835 : *2* : 214.
Lees, Robert.
  A personal communication.
Lindeboom, G. A.
  Hermann Boerhaave—The Man and his Work. London. 1968.
Liston, Robert.
  Ligature of Subclavian Artery. *Med. Times Hosp. Gaz.* 1820 :*16* : 120.
Little, George A.
  Malachi Horan Remembers. Dublin. 1943.
McDowell, R. B.
  Brit. Assoc. for Advancement of Science. A View of Ireland. Dublin. 1957.
MacNalty, Sir Arthur S.
  The British Medical Dictionary. London. 1961.
Macalister, Alexander.
  A Sketch of Anatomy in Ireland. *Dubl. J. med. Sci.* 1884 : *77* : 1.
  James Macartney. London. 1900.
Madden, Thomas More.
  Recent Medical Progress and Celtic Medicine. *Dubl. J. med. Sci.* 1889 : *108* : 430.
Mahaffy, Sir John.
  The Book of Trinity College, Dublin (1591–1891). Belfast. 1892.

Mapother, E. D.
  Lessons from Lives of Irish Surgeons. *Dubl. J. med. Sci.* 1873 :
    56 : 430.
  Great Irish Surgeons. *Irish Monthly.* 1878 : 6 : 12, 88, 159, 221.
  The Medical profession in Ireland and its work. *Dubl. J. Med. Sci.*
    1886 : *82* : 177.
Maxwell, Constantia.
  A History of Trinity College, Dublin (1591–1892). Dublin. 1946.
  Dublin under the Georges (1714–1830). London. 1956.
"Metropolis".
  Anonymous—quoted by Cameron.
Miles, Alexander.
  The Edinburgh School of Medicine before Lister. London. 1918.
Moorhead, T. G.
  A Short History of Sir Patrick Dun's Hospital, Dublin. Dublin.
    1942.
Moore, Norman.
  An Essay on the History of Medicine in Ireland. *St. Bartholomew's*
    Hospital Reports. 1875 : *11* : 145.
Moore, William D.
  Outline of the History of Pharmacy in Ireland. *Dubl. Quart. J.*
    med. Sci. 1848 : 6 : 64.
  Extracts from Records of the Corporation of the Barber–Surgeons
    of Dublin. *Dubl. J. med. Sci.* 1849 : *8* : 232.
Murphy, J. C. J. (Mrs.).
  The Kilkenny Marble Works. *Old Kilkenny Review.* No. 11 : 1949.
O'Halloran, Sylvester.
  A complete treatise on Gangrene and Sphacelus with a new mode
    of amputation. London. 1765.
O'Malley, C. D.
  Andreas Vesalius of Brussels. *Univ. of Calif. Press.* 1964.
Paterson, Robert.
  Memorials of the life of James Syme. Edinburgh. 1874.
Porter, William Henry.
  Observations on the surgical pathology of the larynx and trachea.
    Dublin. 1826.
Power, Sir D'Arcy.
  A short History of St. Bartholomew's Hospital. London. 1923.
Ramsden, Thomas.
  Practical Observations. London. 1811.
Roney, Cusack.
  Quoted by A. Ellis. *Dublin Medical Press.* 1847 : *17* : 59.

Russell, K. F.
British Anatomy (1525–1800). Melbourne, 1963.
Skinner, Henry Alan. Origin of Medical Terms. 2nd Edit. Baltimore.
1961.
Smith, Aquilla.
Contributions to the History of Medicine. *Dubl. J. med. Sci.*
1840 : *17* : 210.
Some account of the origin and early history of the College of
Physicians in Ireland. *Dubl. J. med. Sci.* 1841 : *19* : 81.
Smith, Robert William.
A Treatise on Fractures in the Vicinity of Joints. Dublin. 1847.
Stokes, William.
Observations on the case of the late Abraham Colles. *Dubl.
Quart J. med. Sci.* 1846 : *No. 1* : 303.
Observations on some cases of permanently slow pulse. *Dubl.
Quart J. med. Sci.* 1846 : *No. 2* : 73.
Lectures on Fevers. Edit. J. W. Moore. London. 1874.
Stokes, Sir William.
Work done in Surgery by its Professors in R.C.S.I. *Dubl. J. med.
Sci.* 1887 : *84* : 353.
William Stokes. London. 1898.
Struthers, John.
Anatomical and Physiological Observations. Edinburgh. 1854.
Historical Sketch of the Edinburgh Anatomical School. Edin-
burgh. 1867.
Trevelyan, G. M.
Foreword to Maxwell's History of Trinity College, Dublin.
Dublin. 1946.
Todd, Charles H.
Ligature of Subclavian Artery. *Dubl. Hosp. Reports.* 1822 : *3* :
466.
Underwood, E. Ashworth.
Boerhaave after 300 years. *Br. med. J.* 1968 : *4* : 820.
Widdess, J. D. H.
A History of the Royal College of Physicians in Ireland (1654–
1963). Edinburgh. 1963.
A History of the Royal College of Surgeons in Ireland and its
Medical School. 2nd Edit. Edinburgh. 1967.
Wilde, William R.
History of periodic medical literature in Ireland. *Dubl. Quart. J.
med. Sci.* 1846 : *1* : 1.
Sylvester O'Halloran. *Dubl. Quart. J. med. Sci.* 1848 : *6* : 223.

Wilson, T. G.
  Victorian Doctor. London. 1942.
Wright-St. Clair, R. E.
  Doctors Monro. London. 1964.

(B)   Biographical (Abraham Colles):

Bailey, Hamilton and Bishop, W. J.
  Notable names in Medicine and Surgery. London. 1959.
Benjamin, John A.
  Invest. Urol. 1965 : *3* : 321.
Bettany, G. T.
  Dictionary National Biography. 1887 : *11* : 333.
Biographical Brevities.
  Am. J. Surg. 1930 : *8* : 169.
Biographical Notes.
  Br. J. Surg. 1914 : *11* : 351.
Cameron, Sir Charles A.
  History of the Royal College of Surgeons in Ireland. 2nd Edit.
    Dublin. 1916.
Doescher, T. F.
  Albany med. Ann. 1908 : *29* : 598.
Doolin, William.
  Med. Press and Circular. 1933 : *136* : 71.
  J. Bone Jt. Surg. 1954 : *36* : 132.
  J. Ir. med. Ass. 1955 : *36* : 1.
  Oxf. med. Sch. Gaz. 1958 : *10* : 53.
Dublin University Magazine. 1844 (June). 688.
Editorial.
  J. Amer. med. Ass. 1962 : *179* : 722.
Editorial.
  Rly. Surg. 1897 : *4* : 154.
Gurlt, E. and Hirsch, A.
  Biographisches Lexikon der Hervorrgenden Aerzte. 1885 : *2* : 55.
Hall, D. P.
  Am. J. Surg. 1960 : *99* : 259.
Hunter, R. H.
  Ulster med. J. 1933 : *2* : 133.
Jones, A. R.
  J. Bone Jt. Surg. 1950 : *32* : 126.
Kelly, E. C.
  Med. Class. 1940 : *4* : 1027.

Kirkpatrick, T. Percy C.
History of Dr. Steevens' Hospital, Dublin. Dublin. 1924.
Ir. J. med. Sci. 1931 : *No. 66* : 61.
McDonnell, Robert.
Memoir in Selections from the Works of Abraham Colles. London.
1881.
Peltier, Leonard F.
Surgery—St. Louis. 1954 : *35* : 322.
Power, Sir D'Arcy.
Br. J. Surg. 1921 : *9* : 4.
Russell, K. F.
Aust. N.Z. J. Surg. 1938 : *8* : 115.
Stack, James K.
Surg. Gynec. Obstet. 1936 : *62* : 251.
Studies in Biography.
Intercolon. med. J. Australasia. 1906 : *11* : 105.
Wilson, T. G.
The Practitioner. 1953 : *170* : 407.

Index